P ENELOPE BY
    Museum of Co:
    Centre in Bath ι
She has written several
and is now Joint Editor of *Costume*, the Journal of the
Costume Society. Her particular interest is dress in
nineteenth century literature and she is a Life Member
of the Jane Austen Society.

Jane Austen
Fashion

FASHION AND NEEDLEWORK IN THE
WORKS OF JANE AUSTEN

PENELOPE BYRDE

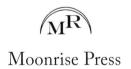

Moonrise Press

Moonrise Press
Ludlow

ISBN 978-0-9539561-3-5

Acknowledgements

I am grateful to several people who kindly assisted in the publication of
this book: Stephen Bird, Patricia Dunlop, Judith Zedner and Jacqueline
Campbell of Bath and North East Somerset Council; Jean Bowden and
Tom Carpenter of Jane Austen's House at Chawton and the late Mr Alwyn
Austen.

Extracts from Jane Austen's works are quoted with the permission of the
Oxford University Press.

Illustrations (numbered by the pages on which they appear) are
reproduced with the kind permission of the following:

Alwyn Austen Esq: 1
Jane Austen's House, Chawton: 15, 31, 32
Bath Reference Library: 5, 9, 21, 26, 27, 28, 30
The Museum of Costume and Fashion Research Centre, Bath (now the
Fashion Museum): 3, 4, 6, 10, 11, 18, 23, 25, 29
Victoria and Albert Museum: 2, 7, 8, 12, 13, 14, 16, 17, 19, 20, 22, 24, 33-36

Contents

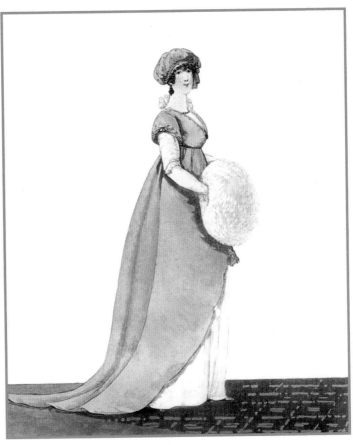

Niklaus von Heideloff, *The Gallery of Fashion*, February 1803

This fashion plate illustrates a blue open-fronted gown and white petticoat, with Elizabethan-style ruff collar of white lace. Turban-shaped cap to match and a large white fur muff.

Preface

THIS BOOK WAS first published in 1979, by the then Bath City Council, in the form of a booklet called *A Frivolous Distinction. Fashion and Needlework in the Works of Jane Austen.* The idea for it arose a few years earlier, during the 1975 bi-centenary of Jane Austen's birth. Celebrations that year – held at places connected with her life, such as Steventon, Chawton and Bath – had included displays of costume, needlework and needlework tools. Some of these items belonged to Jane Austen herself while others were examples which survived from her lifetime; but all were a reminder of the comments she had made both in letters to her sister and in her novels to the fashions and handwork which were popular at that time.

It was felt that a short but detailed study of Jane Austen's comments on this subject might be of value. It is a period which fascinates many people and recent television and film adaptations of the novels have brought her work to an even wider public, eager for information about it. Jane Austen's own viewpoint offers valuable insights into the dress of her time. She tells us not only what clothes were fashionable when she was a young woman, but how they were made, where they were bought, what was worn for special occasions and what her contemporaries thought and felt about their clothes.

A Frivolous Distinction eventually went out of print and might have remained so had it not been for the enthusiasm of David Burnett of Excellent Press who published a new hardback edition in 1999. The text of the original work remained largely unchanged but new illustrations were added and the book was redesigned by Penny Mills. The current paperback edition has been printed by Moonrise Press, Ludlow and I am grateful to Jane Moon for her commitment to keeping *Jane Austen Fashion* in print.

Jane Austen's references to fashion and needlework have been compiled and arranged in six chapters. Each chapter includes a general introduction and discussion of an aspect of dress with quotations from Jane Austen's works. The sources of the quotations are included at the end of the book. There is also a brief guide to the textile terms used by Jane Austen and a short bibliography.

The original spelling and punctuation in quotations from Jane Austen's letters have been preserved. Thus words such as 'ribbon' appears as 'ribband' and 'pleated' is spelt 'plaited' (as was usual in the nineteenth century). Prices are of course in the old currency of pounds, shillings and pence (frequently abbreviated to 's' and 'd' for shillings and pence).

The illustrations have been chosen to complement passages in the text. These include some items of surviving

surviving costume and fashion plates from the period of Jane Austen's life. Many of these come from the collections at the Museum of Costume and Fashion Research Centre in Bath (now the Fashion Museum) but there are also some pieces from Jane Austen's House at Chawton. A number of the fashion plates are taken from *The Gallery of Fashion*, illustrated and published by Niklaus von Heideloff from 1794 to 1803. This was one of the earliest and best English fashion magazines. It is unlikely that Jane or Cassandra Austen would have subscribed to such an expensive magazine (initially it cost three guineas a year) but they might well have seen plates like these on visits to the dressmaker or milliner. The fashion plates are reproduced from collections at the Victoria and Albert Museum, London, the Fashion Research Centre, Bath (now the Fashion Museum) and Bath Reference Library.

Penelope Byrde
2008

CHAPTER ONE

Jane Austen

1775–1817

JANE AUSTEN was born on 16 December 1775 at Steventon Rectory, Hampshire. She was the seventh child of a family of eight children and particularly attached to her sister Cassandra with whom she later corresponded regularly whenever they were separated. Cassandra and Jane were sent away to school for a short time in Oxford and in Southampton, and then to the Abbey School in Reading but until 1801 the family remained at Steventon where the Reverend George Austen was the rector.

During this period Jane Austen wrote her first three novels: *Pride and Prejudice* (originally called *First Impressions*) between October 1796 and August 1797; *Sense and Sensibility* (at first named *Elinor and Marianne*) begun in 1795; and *Northanger Abbey* (originally *Susan*) from 1798 to 1799. None of these was published until later.

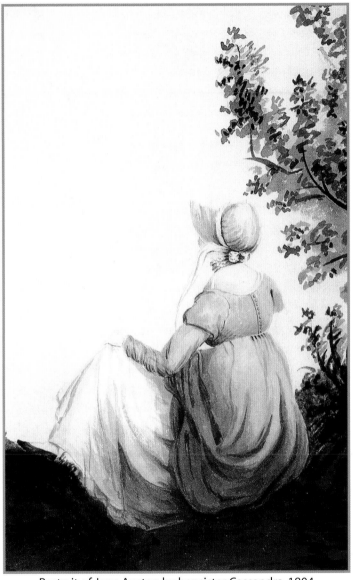

Portrait of Jane Austen by her sister Cassandra, 1804
Private Collection

PREVIOUS PAGE: This charming, informal portrait of Jane Austen shows her sitting on a grassy bank, her face concealed by the deep brim of her bonnet. The low neckline of her gown is filled in with a 'chemisette' with a frilled ruff collar. Her skirt is tucked up over her underskirt or 'petticoat' – a usual precaution at this date when walking.

In 1801 Mr Austen retired and moved with his family to Bath where he died in 1805. The family then moved to Southampton in 1806 and to Chawton, in Hampshire, in 1809.

Between 1809 and 1816 Jane Austen completed three other novels: *Mansfield Park, Emma* and *Persuasion* and she secured the publication of four of her works. *Sense and Sensibility* was the first to be published in 1811; then *Pride and Prejudice* in 1813, *Mansfield Park* in 1814 and *Emma* in 1816. It was not until 1818, after her death, that *Northanger Abbey* and *Persuasion* were published together in one volume. Her other work included a novel called *Lady Susan* (written 1793–4) and two unfinished novels: *The Watsons* (1804) and *Sanditon* (1817).

Jane and Cassandra Austen also spent short periods from home visiting relatives in London or other places such as Lyme Regis in Dorset or Godmersham (the Kent home of her brother Edward). Jane Austen never married and in May 1817 she moved to Winchester for medical treatment. She died there on 18 July at the age of forty-one and was buried in Winchester Cathedral.

Jane Austen makes relatively little reference to contemporary events in her novels although she lived at a period of revolution abroad and war on the Continent. She was fourteen when the French Revolution broke out in 1789 and a young woman during the Napoleonic Wars which culminated in the British naval victory of Trafalgar in 1805 and the battle of Waterloo in 1815. George III was on the throne throughout her lifetime but he became permanently deranged in 1811 and until his death in 1820 his son (the Prince of Wales, later George IV) acted as Regent.

References to contemporary dress are also rather few in the novels of Jane Austen. Most of her heroines do not mention or discuss their clothes in detail, not because they are uninterested in fashion but because it was not considered a suitable or interesting topic for general conversation (any more than it was polite to comment, in public, on other people's personal appearance). Those of her characters who are interested in dress and talk about it to an excessive extent are unfortunately those whose vacant minds or poor manners are underlined by this habit – women such as Miss Steele in *Sense and Sensibility*, Mrs Allen in *Northanger Abbey*, Lydia Bennet in *Pride and Prejudice* and Mrs Elton in *Emma*.

Jane Austen herself had a natural and lively interest in clothes as is evident from her letters to her sister, Cassandra. She enjoyed discussing such matters with her close friends and relatives; no doubt if it had been relevant to the story, characters like Elinor and Marianne Dashwood and Jane and Elizabeth Bennet would have discussed very similar topics with each other. The two heroines who are more absorbed with matters of dress than the others are Fanny Price and Catherine Morland. This was because Fanny was 'young and inexperienced, with small means of choice and no confidence in her own taste – the "how she should be dressed" was a point of painful solicitude.'[1] Catherine, also young and unsure of herself, was anxious about her appearance but the passage in *Northanger Abbey* where she lies awake debating what she should wear for her next ball sums up both male and female attitudes to dress in any period and some of the author's own views on the subject:

> What gown and what head-dress she should wear on the occasion became her chief concern. She cannot be justified in it. Dress is at all times a frivolous distinction, and excessive solicitude about it often destroys its own aim. Catherine knew all this very well; her great aunt had read her a lecture on the subject only the Christmas before; and yet she lay awake ten minutes on Wednesday night debating between her spotted and her tamboured muslin, and nothing but the shortness of the time prevented her buying a new one for the evening. This would have been an error in judgment, great though not uncommon, from which one of the other sex rather than her own, a brother rather than a great aunt might have warned her, for man only can be aware of the insensibility of man towards a new gown. It would be mortifying to the feelings of many ladies, could they be made to understand how little the heart of man is affected by what is costly

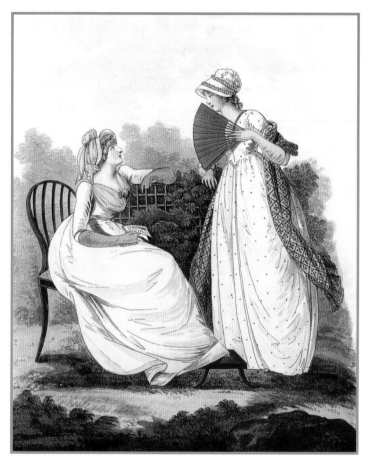

Niklaus von Heideloff, *The Gallery of Fashion*, August 1799

Two young ladies in fashionable day dress. The gowns are almost certainly white cotton and the right-hand dress has a blue spot. The long scarf or shawl may be black net or lace. Other accessories include ribbon-trimmed bonnets, long coloured gloves and a fan. Note: *The Gallery of Fashion*, illustrated and published by Niklaus von Heideloff, was the first English magazine devoted entirely to fashion and the first to have all its plates in colour.

or new in their attire; how little it is biassed by the texture of their muslin, and how unsusceptible of peculiar tenderness towards the spotted, the sprigged, the mull or the jackonet. Woman is fine for her own satisfaction alone. No man will admire her the more, no woman will like her the better for it. Neatness and fashion are enough for the former, and a something of shabbiness or impropriety will be most endearing to the latter. – But not one of these grave reflections troubled the tranquillity of Catherine.[2]

Although the references to dress and needlework are comparatively few in her novels there are many in the letters of Jane Austen and together with those which appear in the novels enough information is provided to give an interesting and often vivid picture of the clothes worn during the period of her lifetime.

CHAPTER TWO

Women's Dress

THE FASHIONS 1775-1817

DURING THE last quarter of the eighteenth century the character of women's dress changed and developed towards the new style which had emerged by the beginning of the nineteenth century and which is usually associated with the Regency period. The stiffness and formality of earlier-eighteenth century dress gradually gave way to something softer, lighter and more informal, or what was considered to be more Romantic. Wide hoop-petticoats were abandoned, to be retained only for Court dress, the waistline gradually began to rise, bodices were filled in with muslin kerchiefs and plain wrapped gowns became fashionable during the 1780s and 1790s. Women's gowns became softer and plainer in both style and decoration as the stiff, richly brocaded or embroidered silks were being replaced by lighter textiles

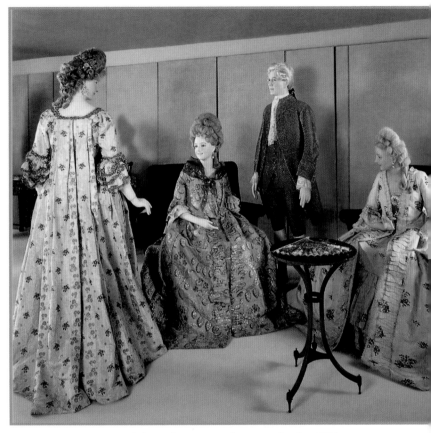

Formal dress for men and women in the 1770s
Museum of Costume, Bath

At the time of Jane Austen's birth, formal clothes for both men and women were made of rich and colourful silks with woven or embroidered patterns and trimmed with gold and silver lace. Lace ruffles were worn by men on their shirt fronts and cuffs, and by women on their sleeves. Powdered hair was usual: in the form of curled wigs for men and towering arrangements of natural hair (greased, powdered and dressed over pads) for women.

such as muslins and gauzes, often of several drifting layers. Light colours were popular. The very tall hair styles of the 1770s eventually collapsed into loose curls while large hats became increasingly fashionable.

The last years of the eighteenth century may be regarded as a transitional period in female fashions but by the beginning of the nineteenth century a new style had evolved and become established. The neo-classical style in contemporary decorative arts extended to female fashion and what was thought of as the revival of the dress of Ancient Greece now took place. Complete simplicity of style, very soft, clinging fabrics, light colours and the most delicate decoration were cultivated. The waistline was placed very high, the bodice was small and plain with short sleeves for evening dress and the skirt was long and flowing. The hair was arranged carefully to appear as natural as possible in shorter, loose curls often held in place with bandeaux or combs.

By about 1810, however, the mood began to change, moving away from the purely Antique towards the Gothic style of decoration. Once established, the form of women's dress with the short waist and column-like silhouette was not easy to alter rapidly but attempts were made to introduce some variety. The bodice became more decorated, greater emphasis was placed on the sleeve, the waistline very gradually began to drop and there was more ornamentation on the hem which encouraged an eventual widening of the skirt.

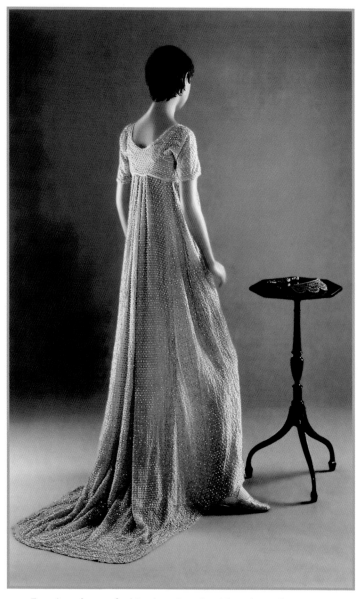

Evening dress of white bead-embroidered muslin, c.1804
Museum of Costume, Bath

Women's Dress in the novels and letters of Jane Austen

Although news of changing fashions was beginning to be spread by the publication of newspapers, periodicals and fashion plates from the end of the eighteenth century, most women still depended on hearing news about clothes from the written or verbal descriptions of friends and relatives visiting or living in London, the large provincial towns, or fashionable resorts such as Bath. In *Pride and Prejudice* the first part of Mrs Gardiner's business on her arrival to stay with the Bennets, 'was to distribute her presents and describe the newest fashions'[1]; and when Jane Bennet returns home from staying with friends she has the same task: her mother, 'Mrs Bennet was doubly engaged, on one hand collecting an account of the present fashions from Jane, who sat some way below her, and on the other, retailing them all to the younger Miss Lucases.'[2] Jane Austen herself frequently exchanged news about the fashions with her sister, especially when visiting London or Bath. She wrote to a friend from London in September 1814: 'I am amused by the present

By the time Jane Austen was in her twenties, dress styles were light, simple and flowing, strongly influenced by the neo-classical taste. Plain white muslin could be embellished for evening wear by different types of white or metal thread embroidery and with beads. However, elegance and restraint were important considerations. Jane Austen's heroine, Emma, 'had herself the highest value for elegance.'

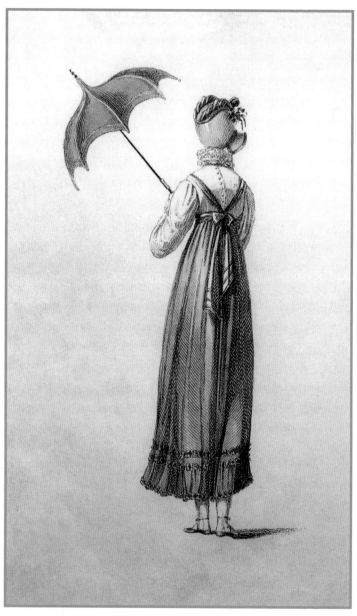

Walking Dress, *Ackermann's Repository of Arts*, August 1814

style of female dress; – the coloured petticoats with braces over the white Spencers & enormous Bonnets upon the full stretch, are quite entertaining. It seems to me a more marked *change* than one has lately seen.'[3]

The spencer was a short jacket cut like the bodice, usually with long sleeves and a high neck. In June 1808 Jane Austen was to write that: 'my kerseymere Spencer is quite the comfort of our Eveng walks.'[4] Spencers could be made of silk as well as woollen cloth.

The pelisse was an over-garment or coat cut on the same lines as the dress, usually with sleeves and fastening at the front. It was an important article of dress at this time and is often mentioned in the novels and letters; it is interesting to see how the author uses it as a simile in *Persuasion*. Captain Wentworth is describing his ship which was an old one by the time he came to command it: 'I knew pretty well what she was, before that day;' he said, 'I had no more discoveries to make, than you would have as to the fashion and strength of any old pelisse, which you had seen lent about among half your acquaintance, ever since you could remember, and which

This fashion plate appeared in the popular English magazine *Ackerrnann's Repository* in August 1814 and illustrates a 'lilac sarsnet petticoat' and 'lilac scarf sash, worn in braces'. Interestingly, Jane Austen wrote about this fashion to a friend from London just a month later, in September 1814: 'I am amused by the present style of female dress; - the coloured petticoats with braces over the white Spencers & enormous Bonnets upon the full stretch, are quite entertaining.'

at last, on some very wet day, is lent to yourself.'[5] In *Mansfield Park* when Fanny Price visited Portsmouth she was not considered worth knowing by the young ladies there for, 'she neither played on the pianoforte nor wore fine pelisses.'[6]

During the eighteenth and early nineteenth century women's gowns could be either open or closed at the front. The gown was usually worn over a petticoat (that is, an underskirt) and in the 1790s might also be worn with a closed robe. Jane Austen's references to petticoats concern underskirts (or underdresses) as main garments rather than items of underclothing. In *Pride and Prejudice* when Elizabeth Bennet walked three miles to visit her sister her appearance was criticised by her friends: 'I hope you saw her petticoat, six inches deep in mud, I am absolutely certain; and the gown which had been let down to hide it, not doing its office.'[7] In December 1798 Jane Austen mentions her intention of turning one of her older gowns into a petticoat.[8]

Concern about sleeves appears in both her letters and novels. Although long sleeves were worn during the day, it was usual in the evening to wear short sleeves with a low-cut neckline. By 1814 long sleeves were beginning to be worn in the evening and Jane Austen seems to have been determined to wear them herself (she was now in her late thirties and, only three years before her death, not in the best of health). 'I wear my gauze gown today', she wrote in March 1814, 'long sleeves & all; I shall see how they succeed, but as yet I have no reason to suppose long sleeves are allowable.' But she goes on to say: 'Mrs Tilson had long sleeves too, & she assured me that they are worn in the evening by many. I was glad

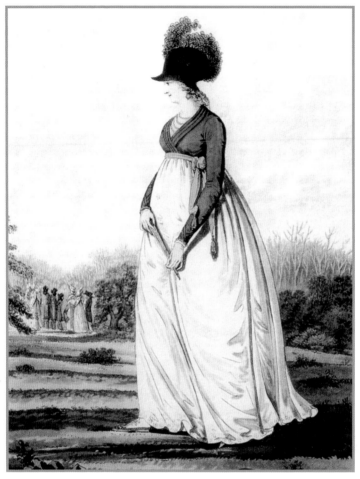

Niklaus von Heideloff, *The Gallery of Fashion*, April 1798

The spencer, which first became fashionable in the 1790s, was a very short jacket worn over the gown to provide extra warmth. Spencers were made of wool or silk, in a wide range of colours, often providing a strong contrast to plain white muslin gowns. 'My kerseymere Spencer is quite the comfort of our Eve[nin]g walks' wrote Jane Austen in 1808.

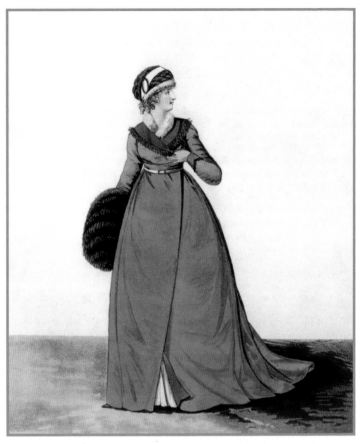

Niklaus von Heideloff, *The Gallery of Fashion*, March 1799

A wrap-over coat or pelisse (probably of silk) in green lined and faced with blue. The shawl collar and cuffs are trimmed with black fringe which may be silk thread or fine beads. Jane Austen mentions trimmings of various kinds, including beads. The edge of the lady's cap and the tippet tucked into her neck are of swansdown. In *Mansfield Park*, when Fanny Price visited Portsmouth, she was not considered worth knowing by the young ladies there, for 'she neither played on the pianoforte nor wore fine pelisses.'

to hear this.'[9] In September she wrote from London that 'long sleeves appear universal, even as Dress.'[10] Mrs Bennet in *Pride and Prejudice* was evidently concerned with the same subject and when her sister visited her from London she confided, 'I am very glad to hear what you tell us, of long sleeves.'[11]

Several of Jane Austen's letters refer to the making of gowns with trains.[12] Evening dresses at this period were usually cut with a fullness at the back to form a small train and we can imagine, in *The Watsons*, how 'Mrs E[dward]'s sattin gown swept along the clean floor of the Ball-room.'[13] In *Northanger Abbey* Isabella Thorpe and Catherine Morland 'pinned up each other's train for the dance.'[14]

Underclothes

The looser, simpler styles of women's dress during the last years of the eighteenth century brought with them more lightly-boned stays or corsets and they began to shrink in size as the bodice of the dress shortened. By the beginning of the nineteenth century the 'Grecian' figure had become fashionable so that clothes were styled to reveal the natural and well-rounded contours of the female figure. Nevertheless many women continued to wear stays and these altered in shape to suit the fashion. In London in September 1813 Jane Austen noted: 'I learnt from Mrs Tickars's young lady [probably a dressmaker's assistant], to my high amusement, that the stays now are not made to force the Bosom up at all; – *that* was a very unbecoming, unnatural fashion. I was really glad to hear that they are not to be worn so much off the shoulders as they were.'[15] (Stays were worn with shoulder straps at this date). As a foundation garment they were an important item for any woman to buy and the following month she writes that her nieces went into Canterbury to try on new stays.[16] The new short-waisted style of women's dresses, so deceptively simple in appearance could, in fact, be very restricting and the tight constriction of the raised waistline round the rib cage extremely uncomfortable.

The chemise or shift, usually made of linen, was worn by all women. Shifts were made at home or bought ready-made. For example, Jane Austen bought six shifts from a travelling salesman in November 1798.[17] New or second-hand shifts were also given to the servants or poor acquaintances by the Austen family.

Jane Austen seems to have had a weakness for stockings and she told Cassandra that she preferred to have only two pairs of a fine quality to three of an inferior sort.[18] The best were made of silk; in April 1811 she bought three pairs 'for a little less than 12./S a pr.'[19] and in September 1813 her niece Fanny was 'very much pleased with the Stockings she has bought of Remmington – Silk at 12S. – Cotton at 4.3. – She thinks them great bargains, but I have not seen them yet'.[20] Apart from silk and cotton, stockings could also be made of wool but the worsted ones she mentions buying were given away to people in need and were doubtless warm and practical rather than elegant. Unlike modern stockings, early-nineteenth century versions were comparatively short, worn over the knee and fastened just below it with garters. Jane Fairfax, in *Emma*, knitted a pair of garters for her grandmother.[21] At night, night-gowns and night-caps were worn. Dressing-gowns were worn over the night-gown or while dressing.

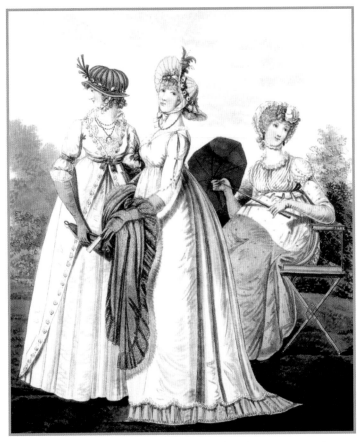

Niklaus von Heideloff, *The Gallery of Fashion*, June 1798

This plate illustrates both types of gown worn at the turn of the nineteenth century: either open at the front and worn over an underskirt or 'petticoat' as it was called, or made in one piece (a 'round gown' with the bodice and skirt being joined by a seam at the waist). Sleeves are elbow length and worn with long gloves. Small parasols with folding handles were fashionable accessories (open on the right, closed and folded on the left). The centre figure carries a black net or lace cloak over her arm.

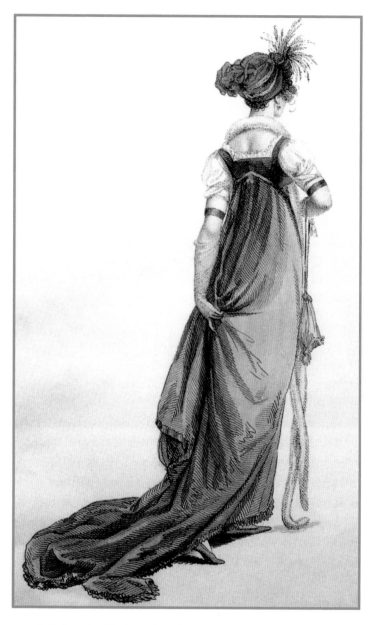

Full dress by Madame Lanchester, *Miroir de la Mode*, 1803

Accessories

Shawls: Shawls of light wool or silk were worn by most women and at the beginning of the nineteenth century the fashion for Indian shawls of cashmere wool soon became widespread. At first, the shawls imported from the East, woven with the traditional pine cone pattern, tended to be rectangular in shape but later they became square. They were more readily available once they were copied and manufactured in textile centres such as Norwich, Paisley and Edinburgh. Lady Bertram in *Mansfield Park* was very anxious to have a shawl from the East: 'William must not forget my shawl, if he goes to the East Indies; and I shall give him a commission for anything else that is worth having. I wish he may go to the East Indies, that I may have my shawl. I think I will have two shawls.'[22] It is evident that shawls could be made of the lightest fabrics and Jane Austen mentions in a letter of April 1805: 'Mary Whitby's turn is actually come to be grown up & have a fine complexion & wear great square muslin shawls.'[23]

Cloaks: Cloaks or mantles at this time were usually wraps of a light material such as the gauzes and lace mentioned in Jane Austen's letters or muslin which

This plate from an English fashion magazine (in spite of its French name) shows that colours other than white could be worn in the evening for 'full dress'. This may be a silk rather than a muslin gown. With it she wears a long boa of swansdown or fur, silk ribbon 'armlet's' and a fashionable handbag or 'reticule'.

Henry Tilney speaks of in *Northanger Abbey*.[24] Often what is called a cloak was a broad scarf with long ends which fell like a stole at the front. Tippets were also worn over the shoulders.

Hats and Caps: On the head hats and bonnets were customary wear out of doors; for married women and ladies in their late twenties onwards caps were worn indoors. The making of caps and trimming of bonnets were carried on to a considerable extent at home and formed an important topic of conversation whenever dress was discussed. Jane Austen herself often comments on the subject. In December 1798 she tells Cassandra: 'I took the liberty a few days ago of asking your Black velvet Bonnet to lend me its cawl, which it very readily did, & by which I have been enabled to give considerable improvement of dignity to my Cap.'[25] Bonnets could be made of any number of different materials apart from straw (chip or strip) such as beaver, velvet, silk, crape, satin, muslin or cloth. For example, in May 1801 Jane wrote: 'My Mother has ordered a new Bonnet, & so have I; – both white chip, trimmed with white ribbon. – I find my straw bonnet looking very much like other peoples & quite as smart. – Bonnets of Cambric Muslin on the plan of L[ad]y Bridges' are a good deal worn, & some of them are very pretty; but I shall defer one of that sort till your arrival.'[26]

In *Pride and Prejudice* Lydia Bennet's frivolous character is illustrated by her attitude to clothes: 'Look here, I have bought this bonnet,' she announces, 'I do not think it is very pretty; but I thought I might as well buy it as not. I shall pull it to pieces as soon as I get home, and see if I can make it up any better.' 'And when her sisters abused it as ugly, she added, with perfect unconcern, "Oh! but there were two or three much uglier in the shop; and when I have bought some prettier-coloured satin to trim it with fresh, I think it will be very tolerable ... I am glad I bought my bonnet, if it is only for the fun of having another bandbox!"'[27]

In the last years of the 1790s a particular fashion for trimming hats with artificial flowers and fruit became widespread and Jane Austen finds herself involved, while staying in Bath, in shopping around for these decorations, though she describes the fashion with some irony. In June 1799 she told Cassandra: 'Flowers are very much worn, & Fruit is still more the thing. – Elizth: has a bunch of Strawberries, & I have seen Grapes, Cherries, Plumbs & Apricots – There are likewise Almonds & raisins, french plumbs & Tamarinds at the Grocers, but I have never seen any of them in hats. – A plumb or green gage would cost three shillings; – Cherries & Grapes about 5 I beleive [sic] – but this is at some of the dearest Shops; – My aunt has told me of a very cheap one near Walcot Church, to which I shall go in quest of something for You.'[28] In her next letter she says: 'Though you have given me unlimited powers concerning Your Sprig, I cannot determine what to do about it, & shall therefore in this & in every other future letter continue to ask you for further directions. – We have been to the cheap Shop, & very cheap we found it, but there are only flowers made there, no fruit – & as I could get 4 or 5 very pretty sprigs of the former for the same money which would procure only one Orleans plumb, in short, could get more for three or four Shillings than I could have means of bringing home, I cannot decide on the fruit till I hear from you again. – Besides, I cannot help thinking that it is more natural to have flowers grow out of the head than fruit.'[29]

Caps, hats and bonnets were also trimmed with ribbon, often brightly coloured like the fashionable poppy-red called 'coquelicot'. Isabella Thorpe in *Northanger Abbey* told Catherine Morland: 'do you know, I saw the prettiest hat you can imagine, in a shop window in Milsom-Street just now – very like yours, only with coquelicot ribbons instead of green; I quite longed for it.'[30]

Veils of net or lace were also worn on bonnets and hats to give extra protection to the face or provide an attractive trimming. The veils hung from the brim to the level of the chin or just covered the eyes.

Caps worn for the evening could also be quite elaborately trimmed like the one Jane Austen was altering in December 1798: 'I still venture to retain the narrow silver round it, put twice round without any bow, & instead of the black military feather shall put in the Coquelicot one, as being smarter; – & besides

A maid, in plain dark gown, apron and cap, helps her mistress to get dressed by adjusting the back lacing of her boned corset. A 'busk' of bone or wood was inserted at the centre front to create a fashionably rigid and upright posture. The corset or 'stays', as they were known at this time, were worn over a linen shift. Long linen drawers were only just coming into use and were considered rather daring.

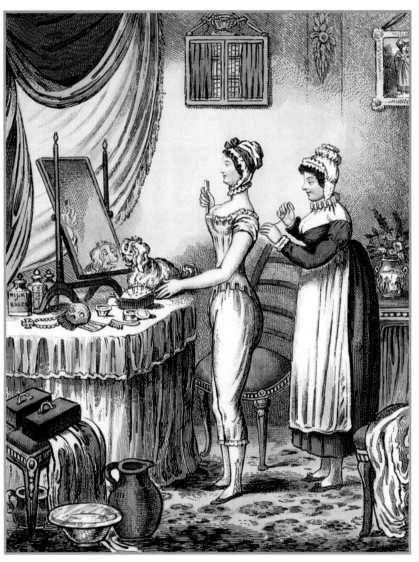

Lady's Toilette, 1810

Coquelicot is to be all the fashion this winter. – After the Ball, I shall probably make it entirely black.' But a little later she adds, 'I have changed my mind, & changed the trimmings of my Cap this morning; they are now such as you suggested; – I felt as if I should not prosper if I strayed from your directions'.[31]

Another cap familiar to us from her letters was a 'Mamalouc' cap she was lent on one occasion and which, she said in January 1799, 'is all the fashion now.'[32] The vogue for Mamalouc (or Mameluk) caps, robes and cloaks had appeared after the battle of the Nile against Napoleon in August 1798. A fashion plate of 1804 illustrating a Mameluk cap shows a white satin turban trimmed with a white ostrich feather.[33] Jane Austen mentions other caps of her own or her nieces' of satin and sarsenet trimmed with lace or flowers.[34]

Footwear: Shoes of the plain, slipper type were worn indoors and for the evening. Jane Austen mentions them of a number of different colours: green, pink, white, black and the exciting blue shoes in *Sanditon*. Mr

Of all costume accessories at this period, the shawl was the most fashionable and desirable item. The finest (and correspondingly most expensive) examples were the genuine cashmere shawls from India. 'Shawls are much worn' said one fashion magazine in 1809, 'they are admirably adapted to the promenade, as they afford, in the throw and arrangement, such fine opportunities for the display of the wearer's taste.'

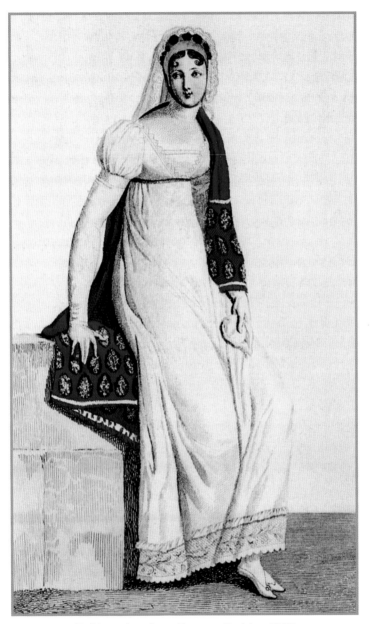

Fashion plate from *Costume Parisien*, 1810

Parker exclaimed: 'civilisation, civilisation indeed! ...
Look at William Heeley's windows. – Blue Shoes and
nankin Boots! – Who would have expected such a sight
at a Shoemaker's in old *Sanditon*! – This is new within
the Month. There was no blue Shoe when we passed this
way a month ago ... Glorious indeed!'[35] These coloured
shoes were not necessarily made of leather; fabrics such
as satin were also used.

In September 1814 Jane Austen wrote to her niece,
Anna, 'your Grandmama desires me to say that she will
have finished your Shoes tomorrow & thinks they will
look very well'.[36] She may have simply been trimming
them because shoes were usually bought from a
shoemaker either ready-made or made to measure. She
mentions buying shoes for her friends and relations[37]
but those with more means would have had their shoes
made for them. Lord Osborne in *The Watsons* begged
'that his Sister might be allow'd to send Emma the
name of her Shoemaker'[38] and in *Mansfield Park* Mary
Crawford told Fanny Price that her friend 'will be at me
for ever about your eyes and your teeth, and how you do
your hair, and who makes your shoes.'[39]

Indoor shoes were certainly not suitable for walking
long distances and concern about footwear appears in
several incidents in the novels. In *Emma*, for example,
Isabella Knightley, worried about returning home
before the snow becomes too thick, says: 'I am not at all
afraid. I should not mind walking half the way. I could
change my shoes, you know, the moment I got home.'
And her husband replies: 'Walk home! – You are prettily
shod for walking home, I dare say. It will be bad enough
for the horses.'[40]

Half-boots for walking or riding were fashionable for women. Emma Woodhouse in *Emma* tries tactfully to fall behind her two companions when out walking by fiddling with the lacing of her half-boot. 'She then broke the lace off short, and dexterously throwing it into a ditch, was presently obliged to entreat them to stop, and acknowledge her inability to put herself to rights so as to be able to walk home in tolerable comfort. "Part of my lace is gone ... Mr Elton, I must beg leave to stop at your house, and ask your housekeeper for a bit of ribband or string, or anything just to keep my boot on."'[41]

Nankin was another fabric used for footwear and in particular for the half-boots mentioned in the two unfinished novels *Sanditon* and *The Watsons*. Nankin was a stout cotton of a brownish-yellow colour named after Nanking, its place of origin. In *The Watsons* Lord Osborne tells Emma Watson: "you should wear half-boots ... Nothing sets off a neat ankle more than a half-boot; nankin galoshed with black [a band of leather running round the lower part above the sole] looks very well – Do not you like Half-boots?" "Yes", replied Emma, "– but unless they are so stout as to injure their beauty, they are not fit for Country walking."[42]

For really wet and muddy weather and especially in the country, it was still the custom for some people to wear pattens. These were over-shoes with wooden soles supported on an iron ring or frame which raised the wearer several inches from the ground and made a noise on any hard surface. Jane Austen mentions the 'ceaseless clink of pattens'[43] among the many noises of Bath which Anne Elliot found so trying in *Persuasion*. Edward Austen-Leigh remembered his aunts Jane and Cassandra wearing pattens although by the end of the eighteenth century he says they were 'banished from good society, and employed only in menial work.'[44] At *Northanger Abbey* Catherine Morland noted that 'wherever they went, some pattened girl stopped to curtsey.'[45]

Parasols and umbrellas: Other accessories for protection against the weather were parasols and umbrellas. Small parasols, often matching the gown or pelisse in colour or material were fashionable in the summer. In May 1801 Jane Austen went out for a walk in Bath and was concerned that her friend should be 'without any parasol or any shade to her hat.'[46] In *Sanditon* Mr Parker brushed aside his wife's concern for their children spending too long in the garden in the sun: 'you can get a Parasol at Whitby's for little Mary at any time, or a large Bonnet at Jebb's – and as for the Boys, I must say I would rather them run about in the Sunshine than not.' Mrs Parker replies: 'I will get Mary a little Parasol, which will make her as proud as can be. How Grave she will walk about with it, and fancy herself quite a little Woman.'[47]

Plain white muslin dresses were set off by brightly-coloured accessories such as parasols and umbrellas (usually green), scarves, gloves and bonnets made of straw or fabric trimmed with ribbon. Fashionable bonnets had deep, funnel-shaped brims. When Catherine Morland arrived at *Northanger Abbey* a 'sudden scud of rain ... fixed all her thoughts on the welfare of her new straw bonnet'.

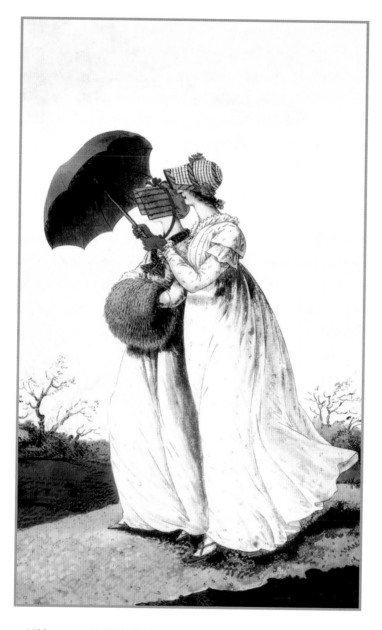

Niklaus von Heideloff, *The Gallery of Fashion*, November 1801

Several references to umbrellas in both the novels and letters seem to imply Jane Austen's belief that it rained a great deal in Bath; indeed, in *Persuasion* Captain Wentworth tells Anne Elliot: 'Though I came only yesterday, I have equipped myself properly for Bath already, you see' (pointing to a new umbrella).[48] On the other hand, in a town like Bath which was small enough to go almost everywhere on foot, an umbrella was a convenient alternative to using a carriage or sedan chair for protection and transport when it rained. And, since part of the 'cure' here was to take regular walks, walking sticks and umbrellas were recognised accessories to spa dress.

Muffs and gloves: Large muffs were fashionable during the early years of the nineteenth century and often matched the tippet or cape. Otherwise the hands were kept warm by gloves or mittens which were an important dress accessory especially for the evening. Gloves were made of leather or other materials such as silk and could be hand-knitted (Mrs Austen apparently enjoyed making them very much).[49]

Jane Austen seems to have been particular about both gloves and stockings she bought. In October 1798 she told Cassandra: 'I have unpacked the Gloves & placed yours in your drawer. – Their colour is light & pretty, & I beleive [sic] exactly what we fixed on.'[50] In May 1812 she was pleased to write that: 'I was very lucky in my gloves, got them at the first shop I went to, though I went into it rather because it was near than because it looked at all like a glove shop, & gave only four Shillings for them; – upon hearing which, everybody at Chawton will be hoping & predicting that they cannot be good for anything, and their worth certainly remains to be proved, but I think they look very well.'[51]

Fans: Fans were used during the evening at assemblies and dances. Jane Austen mentions her own 'white fan'[52] and the fans of two of her heroines, Fanny Price[53] and Catherine Morland.[54]

Bags and Purses: Necessary items such as a fan, scent bottle or pocket handkerchief were carried in a small bag or reticule which was often circular or lozenge-shaped. Mrs Elton in *Emma* had a purple and gold reticule or 'ridicule' in which she had carried a letter.[55] A fashionable form of purse for carrying money at this time was the so-called Stocking, Miser's or Ring purse, long and narrow in shape, with an opening in the centre, two rings to close it and ornaments at either end. Many of these were knitted, netted or crocheted and making purses was a popular pastime. Mr Bingley in *Pride and Prejudice*, in fact, considered netting a purse was a female 'accomplishment'.[56]

Jewellery: Jewellery and ornaments were worn a good deal during this period, and hair ornaments were fashionable. In *Emma*, Frank Churchill was pleased that his fiancée was to be given all his aunt's jewels: "they are to be new set. I am resolved to have some in an ornament for the head. Will it not be beautiful in her dark hair?"[57] In *Northanger Abbey* Eleanor Tilney was seen at a ball with 'white beads round her head.'[58]

Other mention is made of bracelets, rings, necklaces, pendants, earrings and brooches. In two instances,

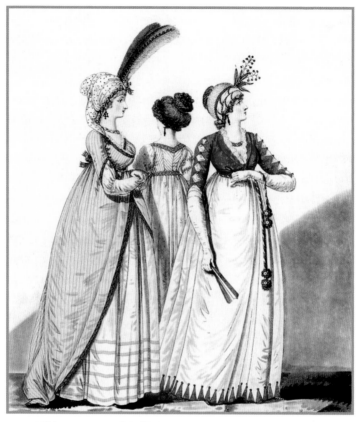

Niklaus von Heideloff, *The Gallery of Fashion*, April 1798

The elaborate head-dresses in this plate suggest that these clothes are for more formal, evening wear. Tall feathers were fashionable in the late 1790s. In *Northanger Abbey*, when Catherine Morland and Mrs Allen attended their first, very crowded ball at the Bath Assembly Rooms, 'they saw nothing of the dancers but the high feathers of some of the ladies'. Artificial flowers and fruit were another fashionable trimming but Jane Austen wrote: 'I cannot help thinking that it is more natural to have flowers grow out of the head than fruit.'

items of jewellery play an important part in the plot of the novels: the ring worn by Edward Ferrars in *Sense and Sensibility* and the amber cross from Sicily which Fanny Price is given by her brother William in *Mansfield Park*. Unfortunately William had not been able to afford a gold chain as well and Fanny wore it on a piece of ribbon, but she did not feel this would be grand enough for her first ball 'in the midst of all the rich ornaments which she supposed all the other young ladies would appear in.'[59] However, both a friend, Mary Crawford, and her cousin Edmund, came to her rescue. Mary Crawford produced a small trinket-box containing several gold chains and asked her to choose one; Fanny took a necklace of gold 'prettily worked' though she would have preferred a longer and plainer chain more adapted for her purpose.[60] As it turned out, the chain would not go through the ring of the cross whereas the present of 'a plain gold chain, perfectly simple and neat' in 'all the niceness of jeweller's packing' from Edmund fitted exactly and was more to Fanny's taste.[61] In the end she wore both to cause no offence. Fanny's amber cross must inevitably be compared with the topaz crosses given to Jane and Cassandra Austen in May 1801 by their brother Charles, who, like William Price, was in the navy. 'He has been buying gold chains & Topaze crosses for us; – he must be well scolded.'[62] (These crosses are still in existence and belong to the Jane Austen Society. They are on display at Jane Austen's House in Chawton).

Also based on reality was the jeweller's shop, Gray's, in Sackville Street, London where in *Sense and Sensibility* 'Elinor was carrying on a negociation for the exchange of a few old-fashioned jewels of her mother.'[63] Her brother, Mr John Dashwood, met Elinor there by chance but carefully explained his financial circumstances in order 'to do away with the necessity of buying a pair of ear-rings for each of his sisters, in his next visit at Gray's.'[64]

Pearl necklaces were worn by those who could afford them. The pretentious Mrs Elton in *Emma* was pleased to note: 'I see very few pearls in the room except mine'[65] and in *Northanger Abbey* 'there was a very beautiful set of pearls ... that Miss Tilney has got now, for they were put by for her when her mother died.'[66]

Less expensive ornaments and trinkets could also be purchased and in fact the circulating libraries during the late-eighteenth and early-nineteenth century dealt not only in books but in other commodities such as these. In *Sanditon* Charlotte Heywood went 'to buy new Parasols, new Gloves, & new Brooches, for her sisters and herself at the Library' and there she found the various goods very tempting but wisely 'turned from the Drawers of rings & Brooches, repressed farther solicitation & paid for what she bought.'[67] Lydia Bennet, also away from home, wrote to her family that she had just been to the library 'where she had seen such beautiful ornaments as made her quite wild.'[68]

Hairdressing: Caroline Austen writing about her Aunt Jane recalled that: 'she always wore a cap – Such was the custom with ladies who were not quite young -– at least of a morning – but I never saw her without one, to the best of my remembrance either morning or evening.'[69] As early as 1798 when Jane Austen was twenty-three she was telling her sister: 'I have made myself two or three caps to wear of evenings since I came home, and they save me a world of torment as to hair-dressing, which at present gives me no trouble beyond washing and brushing, for my long hair is always plaited up out of sight, and my short hair curls well enough to want no papering. I have had it cut lately by Mr Butler [a hairdresser from Basingstoke].'[70] It was fashionable to wear the hair short at the front and it could be curled with the use of papers.

Most ladies had their hair dressed by either a maid or a professional hairdresser, especially for going out in the evening. While staying with her brother's family at Godmersham Park in Kent Jane Austen had her hair dressed by a Mr Hall who came to the house both to do the ladies' hair and give instruction to her sister-in-law's maid. Mr Hall, she told Cassandra: 'charged Eliz:th 5s for every time of dressing her hair, & 5s for every lesson to Sace [the Lady's-maid] ... Towards me he was as considerate, as I had hoped for, from my relationship to you, charging me only 2s 6d for cutting my hair, tho' it was as thoroughly dress'd after being cut for Eastwell [Park, a neighbouring house in Kent], as it had been for the Ashford Assembly.'[71] Some years later in September 1813 she again mentioned Mr Hall who 'was very punctual yesterday, & curled me out at a great rate. I thought it looked hideous, and longed for a snug cap instead, but my companions silenced me by their admiration. I had only a bit of velvet round my head. I did not catch cold however.'[72] A lock of Jane Austen's hair is still to be seen at her house in Chawton.

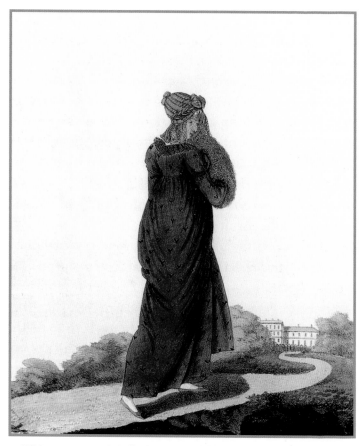

Niklaus von Heideloff, *The Gallery of Fashion*, November 1800

This blue and red patterned garment is likely to be a pelisse (or overcoat) rather than a gown as the lady is walking out of doors. Even for outdoor wear shoes were light and slipper-like. Jane Austen mentions blue shoes in her unfinished novel, *Sanditon*. Large fur muffs were fashionable at this time, as were lace veils attached to the brim of hats or bonnets (to shield the face). It is to this kind of veil that Mrs Elton in *Emma* is referring when she hears of 'very little white satin, very few lace veils' at Emma's wedding.

Cosmetics: Cosmetics were not usually worn but some ladies used rouge and Sir Walter Elliot in *Persuasion* felt that the elderly Lady Russell might benefit from this: 'Morning visits are never fair by women at her time of life, who make themselves up so little. If she would only wear rouge, she would not be afraid of being seen', he remarked.[73]

Sir Walter Elliot, himself an extremely vain man, set great importance on personal appearance and fancied himself an expert on the subject. His daughter Elizabeth once remarked: 'Freckles do not disgust me so very much as they do him: I have known a face not materially disfigured by a few, but he abominates them. You must have heard him notice Mrs Clay's freckles.'[74] On his recommendation Mrs Clay used Gowland's Lotion and he was convinced of its success. Gowland's was a lotion used widely at this time and was described in an advertisement of 1814 as 'the most pleasant and effective remedy for all complaints to which the Face and Skin are liable.'[75] Sir Walter Elliot also found it hard to believe that his second daughter Anne's improved looks were not the result of her using Gowland's Lotion – he thought her 'less thin in her person, in her cheeks; her skin, her complexion, greatly improved – clearer, fresher. Had she been using anything in particular?' 'No, nothing.' 'Merely Gowland', he supposed, 'No, nothing at all.' 'Ha! he was surprised at that;' and added, 'Certainly you cannot do better than continue as you are; you cannot be better than well; or I should recommend Gowland, the constant use of Gowland, during the spring months.'[76]

Many women however liked lavender water as a scent and in *Northanger Abbey* Catherine Morland, concerned about her friend Eleanor, 'obliged her to be seated, rubbed her temples with lavender-water, and hung over her with affectionate solicitude.'[77] In January 1801 Jane asked Cassandra Austen to buy a friend 'two bottles of Steele's Lavender Water when you are in Town, provided you should go to the Shop on your own account.'[78]

The Well-dressed Woman

Although Jane Austen gives us little information about the personal appearance of most of her heroines it seems certain they would always have been suitably and attractively dressed. Her highest praise is always for 'elegance', and this was undoubtedly a contemporary ideal. Jane Fairfax in *Emma*, for example, 'was very elegant, remarkably elegant; and she [Emma] had herself the highest value for elegance.'[79] With Mrs Elton, on the other hand: 'she suspected there was no elegance; – ease but not elegance . . . neither feature, nor air, nor voice, nor manner, were elegant.'[80] Eleanor Tilney in *Northanger Abbey* was perhaps the best-dressed of Jane Austen's female characters: her air, 'though it had not all the decided pretention, the resolute stilishness of Miss Thorpe's, had more real elegance.'[81] As with Emma Woodhouse, the girls whom Jane Austen wishes to be admired in her novels undoubtedly all had 'no taste for finery or parade.'[82]

Not only elegance but propriety in dress was the mark of a lady. When Fanny Price in *Mansfield Park*

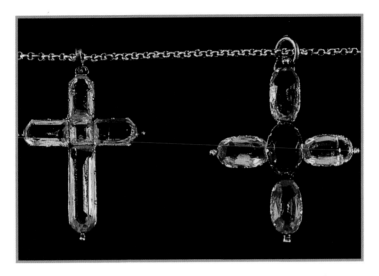

Topaz crosses given to Jane and Cassandra Austen by their brother Charles

In May 1801 Jane wrote to Cassandra that their brother Charles had been 'buying Gold chains & Topaze Crosses for us' with his prize money from the Navy – 'he must be well scolded'. These were probably the inspiration for Fanny Price's amber cross in *Mansfield Park*, brought her from Sicily by her brother William, who like Charles Austen was in the Navy. The topaz crosses are on display at Jane Austen's House in Chawton.

appears for her first ball, her uncle 'saw with pleasure the general elegance of her appearance and her being in remarkably good looks. The neatness and propriety of her dress was all that he would allow himself to commend in her presence, but upon her leaving the

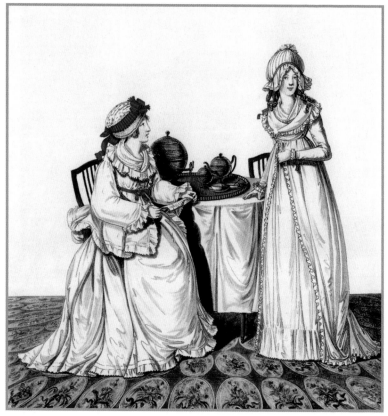

Niklaus von Heideloff, *The Gallery of Fashion*, November 1794

These two ladies are in 'morning dress': informal, easy-fitting garments worn at home in the early part of the day before getting properly dressed. Morning dress was invariably white and could be trimmed with white, open-work embroidery. Married and older women always wore caps indoors.

room again soon afterwards, he spoke of her beauty with very decided praise.'[83]

Jane Austen considered that 'neatness and fashion' were all that men looked for in women's dress[84] and it is clear that she herself had a regard for tidiness and freshness. Caroline Austen recalled that her aunts Jane and Cassandra 'were particularly neat, and they held all untidy ways in great disesteem.'[85] Commenting on her two sisters-in-law in December 1798 Jane said: 'Mary [who had recently had a baby] does not manage matters in such a way as to make me want to lay in myself. She is not tidy enough in her appearance; she has no dressing-gown to sit up in ... Elizabeth was really a pretty object with her nice clean cap put on so tidily and her dress so uniformly white and orderly.'[86] In this instance, Jane Austen's preference for tidiness coincided with current fashion and the popularity of simple, light-weight and light-coloured gowns. Disorderly dress was also disapproved, for instance, by Miss Bingley in *Pride and Prejudice* when she criticised Elizabeth Bennet's appearance after her long walk to Netherfield: 'why must she be scampering about the country, because her sister had a cold? Her hair, so untidy, so blowsy!'[87]

CHAPTER THREE

The Making and Care of Clothes

Dressmaking

WOMEN'S CLOTHES at this period were not, as a rule, bought ready-made (although Jane Austen does mention ready-made cloaks on sale in Alton, Hampshire[1]). Garments such as gowns, pelisses or spencers, which required fitting, were either made to order by a dressmaker or made up at home by ladies themselves and their servants. Similarly, various accessories were supplied by milliners and shoemakers, but caps, hats and bonnets were frequently trimmed at home.

During the eighteenth century the seamstress or dressmaker who made women's gowns was usually known as a 'mantua-maker', the mantua referring to a type of gown which became fashionable at the end of the seventeenth century. The term continued to be used until the middle of the nineteenth century some time

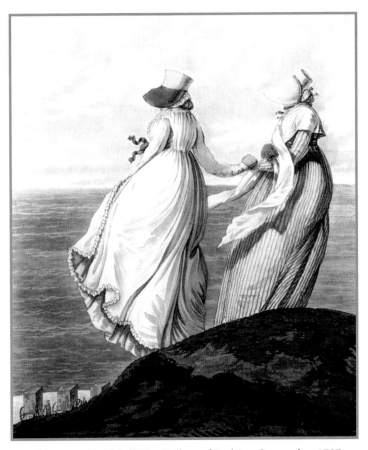

Niklaus von Heideloff, *The Gallery of Fashion*, September 1797

Dresses of the kind shown here were usually made to measure by a professional dressmaker, although most women were able to alter and trim their own clothes. 'I cannot determine what to do about my new Gown,' wrote Jane Austen in 1798, 'I wish such things were to be bought ready made.' This plate illustrates fashionable seaside wear. Jane Austen visited Lyme Regis and mentions bathing there in September 1804. Ladies changed and entered the sea from bathing machines of the kind seen here on the left.

after the mantua went out of fashion and it appears once or twice in Jane Austen's work. In the cancelled chapter of *Persuasion* Admiral Croft is very anxious that Anne Elliot should visit his wife and assures her that she is 'quite alone, nobody but her mantuamaker with her, and they have been shut up together this half-hour, so it must be over soon.' 'Her mantuamaker! Then I am sure my calling now would be most inconvenient.'[2] This passage illustrates the role of the professional dressmaker who would come to the house to receive instructions and take fittings for garments to be made. Alternatively, visits might be made by the customer to the dressmaker; Jane Austen frequently mentions in her letters taking material to be made up into gowns and talks of more than one dressmaker by name. For example, Miss Burton, a London dressmaker, made pelisses for Jane and Cassandra in April 1811. 'Our Pelisses are 17/S each', she wrote, '– she charges only 8/ for the making, but the Buttons seem expensive; – *are* expensive, I might have said – for the fact is plain enough.'[3]

Even when made by the professional dressmaker, the style and construction of a garment were largely dependent on the choice and direction of the customer who would also choose the material. Isabella Thorpe, for instance, asked Catherine Morland in *Northanger Abbey:* 'how do you like my gown? I think it does not look amiss; the sleeves were entirely my own thought.'[4] As a result, the making of any new gown involved some considered planning and it must, at times, have seemed troublesome to make frequent decisions of this kind. Complaining to her sister in December 1798 Jane Austen wrote: 'I cannot determine what to do about my new Gown; I wish such things were to be bought ready made. – I have some hopes of meeting Martha [a friend] at the Christening at Deane next Tuesday, & shall see what she can do for me. – I want to have something suggested which will give me no trouble of thought or direction.'[5] Usually, however, she expresses a natural interest in new clothes. In the same letter, referring to the purchase of a new muslin gown she says: '*I* am determined to buy a handsome one whenever I can, & I am so tired & ashamed of half my present stock, that I even blush at the sight of the wardrobe which contains them.'[6]

At home, dressmaking was undertaken by many ladies themselves and sewing was also done by the maids. In *Mansfield Park*, for instance, Lady Bertram's maid 'was rather hurried in making up a new dress for her'[7] and in *Emma*, Mr Woodhouse speaks of a servant, Hannah, who comes to the house to do needlework.[8]

Jane Austen's nephew in his *Memoir* recalled of his aunt that 'some of her merriest talk was over clothes which she and her companions were making, sometimes for themselves, and sometimes for the poor.'[9] Where her own clothes were concerned, her dressmaking efforts tended towards the alteration or trimming of various garments, such as the gauze gown of which she 'lowered the bosom especially at the corners, & plaited black sattin ribbon round the top.'[10] Jane and Cassandra do not appear to have made their own gowns; for example, from Bath in May 1801 she told Cassandra: 'I will engage Mrs Mussell as you desire. She made my dark gown very well & may therefore be trusted I hope with Yours – but she does not always succeed with lighter Colours. – My white one I was obliged to alter a good deal.'[11]

Some letters to her sister contain minute details of the intended construction of a new gown[12] and her remarks quite often express an awareness of changing fashions, especially when staying in London or at their brother's large country house, Godmersham Park in Kent. In January 1809 she wrote to Cassandra who was visiting Godmersham: 'I can easily suppose that your six weeks here will be fully occupied, were it only in lengthening the waist of your gowns.'[13] Fashion illustrations of this date reflect attempts to lengthen the bodice by a few inches, although it was to be a long time before the waistline returned to its natural level. Several years later, in 1813, when skirt hems were becoming wider and more ornamented, she wrote from Godmersham herself to encourage Cassandra to alter her gowns: 'Miss Chapman' , she says, 'had a double flounce to her gown. – You really must get some flounces. Are not some of your large stock of white morn'g gowns just in a happy state for a flounce, too short?'[14]

Other items such as caps for herself, shirts and cravats for male relatives, baby clothes, shifts and other items for the poor were certainly made at home by Jane Austen and her family. The custom of making clothes for the poor was quite general; in *Mansfield Park* Mrs Norris tells Fanny: 'if you have no work of your own, I can supply you from the poor-basket.'[15]

Mrs Norris also supervised the making of special costumes for the amateur theatricals which were to be staged by the young people in the family. In particular she

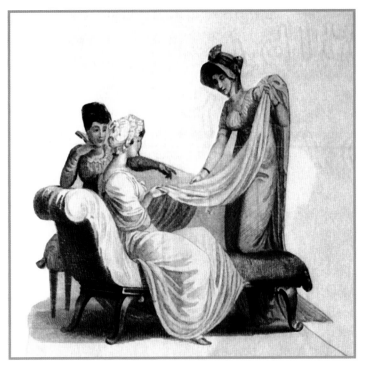

The Most Fashionable Dresses for the Year.
The English Ladies' Pocket Book, 1807

Buying dress fabrics and having them made up into garments were two separate operations at this time. Materials were expensive and needed to be chosen with care – especially muslins which did not always wash or wear well (as both Jane Austen and some of her characters make a point of mentioning). Although there were only four natural fibres in use (wool, silk, linen and cotton) there was great variety in the weight, texture and patterning of dress fabrics to suit each season of the year.

was engaged in making a blue suit and pink satin cloak for Mr Rushworth in his role of Count Cassel in *Lovers' Vows* and complained to Fanny: 'I have been slaving myself till I can hardly stand, to contrive Mr Rushworth's cloak without sending for any more satin; and now I think you may give me your help in putting it together. – There are but three seams, you may do them in a trice.'[16]

In *Northanger Abbey* even Eleanor Tilney, who was well-off and elegant, appears to have done a little of her own dressmaking. Her brother, Henry, tells Catherine Morland that muslin can always be turned to some account: 'I have heard my sister say so forty times, when she has been extravagant in buying more than she wanted, or careless cutting it into pieces.'[17]

Jane Austen mentions on more than one occasion in her letters the length of seven yards to be purchased for a gown for her mother, although in January 1801 she asks Cassandra to buy: 'Seven yards for my mother, seven yards and a half for me' as, she says, she is a taller woman.[18] Writing from London in April 1811 she told her sister that she was tempted, in a linendraper's shop 'by a pretty coloured muslin, & bought 10 yds of it, on the chance of your liking it.'[19] She often refers in her letters to buying 'a gown' but by this she means the standard length of material required to make one and not a garment itself. Ready to wear gowns were not available for sale at this time, except through the second hand market.

Printed paper dressmaking patterns were also not in common use at this date but it is evident that both old and new garments were copied or used as patterns themselves. In January 1801 Jane wrote to Cassandra at Godmersham that 'Mary … will be much obliged to you if you can bring her the pattern of the Jacket & Trowsers, or whatever it is, that Eliz:th's boys wear when they are first put into breeches – ; or if you could bring her an old suit itself she would be very glad, but that I suppose is hardly do-able.'[20] In *Emma* Harriet Smith talks of her 'pattern gown' which she has left at Emma's house.[21] One new or particularly fashionable garment might serve as the pattern for several others and in *Sense and Sensibility* the Misses Steele took patterns from some of Lady Middleton's elegant new dresses.[22] In a letter of January 1807 Jane Austen mentions to her sister that a certain Mrs Dickson had desired Mrs Francis Austen (Jane's sister-in-law who was expecting a baby and with whom she was staying) 'not to provide herself with a christening dress, which is exactly what her young correspondent wanted; and she means to defer making any of the caps as long as she can, in hope of having Mrs D's present in time to be serviceable as a pattern.'[23] Again, in 1813 Jane Austen and her niece have been buying new caps for themselves but she says: 'Fanny is out of conceit with hers already; she finds that she has been buying a new cap without having a new pattern, which is true enough.'[24]

Since procuring and taking new patterns involved a certain effort they were naturally quite highly valued and Jane wryly told Cassandra in June 1799: 'I am quite pleased with Martha & Mrs Lefroy for wanting the pattern of our Caps, but I am not so well pleased with Your giving it to them.'[25]

From the evidence of her letters it appears that women's clothes were altered frequently to vary the style and provide the maximum amount of wear. This was partly because dress fabrics were still expensive to buy. Her nephew in his *Memoir of Jane Austen* said that as a child, her brother Francis Austen's 'first cloth suit was made from a scarlet habit, which, according to the fashion of the time, had been his mother's usual morning dress.'[26]

Textiles and Decoration

Selecting or buying fabrics for new clothes was an important aspect of shopping. Very often friends or relations visiting London or other towns were commissioned to make purchases for those left at home. Jane Austen's letters and novels provide some interesting information about the textiles fashionable during the period. Most frequently mentioned are the various muslins which were, of course, at the height of fashion during the late-eighteenth and early-nineteenth century, having superseded the heavier silks worn earlier.

Muslins, originally imported from India, were subsequently produced in England and Scotland. The term muslin covers many varieties of fine, delicately woven cottons which could be plain, embroidered, or with a woven pattern, of different textures and a wide range of colours. In the passage already mentioned (in Chapter 1), Catherine Morland, the heroine of *Northanger Abbey,* wondering what to wear for her next ball, 'lay awake ten minutes on Wednesday night debating between her spotted and her tamboured muslin', and the author went on to observe that 'it would be mortifying to the feelings of many ladies, could they be made to understand how little the heart of man ... is biassed by the texture of their muslin, and how unsusceptible of peculiar tenderness towards the spotted, the sprigged, the mull or the jackonet.'[27] Henry Tilney, like most other men, was probably indifferent to the finer details of female dress but muslins were such an important topic of conversation amongst ladies in general that he enters humorously but not unkindly, into a discussion with Mrs Allen on the subject. She had told Catherine that the material for her dress had cost but nine shillings a yard.

'...that is exactly what I should have guessed it, madam', said Mr Tilney, looking at the muslin.

'Do you understand muslins, sir?'

'Particularly well; I always buy my own cravats, and am allowed to be an excellent judge; and my sister has often trusted me in the choice of a gown. I bought one for her the other day, and it was pronounced to be a prodigious bargain by every lady who saw it. I gave but five shillings a yard for it, and a true Indian muslin.'

Mrs Allen was quite struck by his genius. 'Men commonly take so little notice of those things,' said she: 'I can never get Mr Allen to know one of my gowns from another. You must be a great comfort to your sister, sir.'

'I hope I am, madam.'

'And pray, sir, what do you think of Miss Morland's gown?'

'It is very pretty, madam,' said he, gravely examining it; 'but I do not think it will wash well; I am afraid it will fray.'[28]

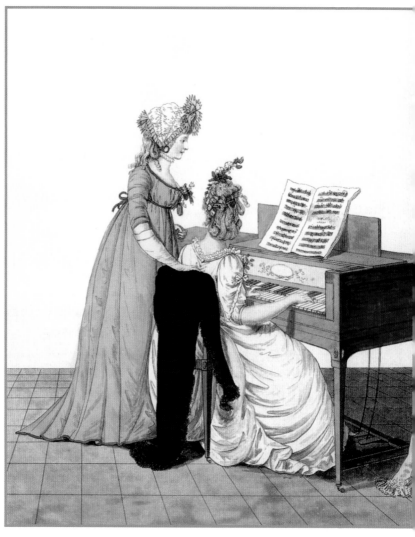

Niklaus von Heideloff, *The Gallery of Fashion*, July 1796

Muslins could vary considerably in quality and might well prove unsatisfactory on occasion. While in Bath in June 1799 Jane Austen 'had no difficulty in getting a muslin veil for half a guinea, & not much more in discovering afterwards that the Muslin was thick, dirty & ragged ... I changed it consequently as soon as I could.'[29]

New fashions in dress textiles had brought several results. The lighter fabrics such as cotton, cambric and muslin had imposed their own character on women's dress and contributed to the softer, lighter, flowing styles. Furthermore these fabrics would wash easily, unlike the elaborate dress silks of the earlier eighteenth century which had to be cleaned in other ways. It now became possible to indulge quite freely the fashion for white or light-coloured gowns which were inspired by classical drapery. White gowns were soon to become the symbol of elegance, refinement and propriety. Eleanor Tilney in *Northanger Abbey*, apparently a model of fashionable and elegant dressing, always wore white.[30] In *Mansfield Park* Fanny Price is worried about appearing over-dressed but her cousin Edmund Bertram assures her that: 'a woman can never be too fine while she is all in white. No, I see no finery about you; nothing but what is perfectly proper.'[31] White was customary for formal morning dress and in the evening; in May 1801

Although white was the most fashionable colour at this period, other plain colours could be worn. Jane Austen mentions several different coloured gowns of her own. However, white gowns were considered correct and refined, especially in the evening.

Jane Austen writes from Bath: 'I like my dark gown very much indeed, colour, make & everything. – I mean to have my new white one made up now, in case we should go to the [Assembly] rooms again next Monday.'[32]

However well muslin might wash it was, nevertheless, not very practical to wear light-coloured gowns, as Mrs Allen complained in *Northanger Abbey:* 'open carriages are nasty things. A clean gown is not five minutes wear in them. You are splashed getting in and getting out.'[33] White gowns could only really be indulged in by those with means and leisure; they were certainly a mark of gentility but might also be considered unsuitable in certain circumstances. In May 1801 Jane Austen wrote from Bath of a Mrs and Miss Holder: 'It is the fashion to think them both very detestable, but they are so civil, & their gowns look so white and so nice (which by the bye my Aunt thinks an absurd pretension in this place) that I cannot utterly abhor them.'[34] In *Mansfield Park* the officious Mrs Norris commends a housekeeper who 'turned away two housemaids for wearing white gowns.'[35]

During the day more practical, coloured gowns could be worn. Discussing her clothes with Cassandra in January 1801 Jane wrote: 'I shall want two new coloured gowns for the summer, for my pink one will not do more than clear me from Steventon. I shall not trouble you, however, to get more than one of them, and that is to be a plain brown cambric muslin, for morning wear; the other, which is to be a plain very pretty yellow and white cloud, I mean to buy in Bath.'[36] Isabella Thorpe in *Northanger Abbey* wrote to her friend Catherine Morland: 'I wear nothing but purple now: I know I look hideous in it, but no matter

– it is your dear brother's favourite colour.'[37] A Miss Fletcher, Jane Austen wrote from Kent in September 1796, 'wore her purple Muslin, which is pretty enough, tho' it does not become her complexion.'[38]

Muslin was an important and fashionable textile not only for gowns but also for a number of other garments such as neckerchiefs or fichus (the 'handkerchiefs' or 'neck handkerchiefs' which Jane Austen refers to), to tuck into the bodice of a gown; for caps, aprons, shawls, veils and even bonnets. As Henry Tilney pointed out, 'muslin always turns to some account or other; Miss Morland will get enough out of it for a handkerchief, or a cap, or a cloak. Muslin can never be said to be wasted.'[39]

Heavier linens, or cottons (such as calico and dimity) were also used and other textiles were undoubtedly necessary for warmth. Gowns and other garments continued to be made of silks and satins. Sarsenet, a type of light silk was particularly popular and there are frequent references to this fabric in contemporary fashion periodicals. Bonnets and pelisses could be made of velvet. Woollen cloth was also worn and Jane Austen mentions morning gowns of 'stuff' which were warm and comfortable but not particularly elegant.[40] She and some of her characters also have a poor opinion of flannel as an attractive textile and this was quite often worn for warm under-garments.

The plainer, softer materials which were now fashionable gave more scope for decoration than the richly-patterned silks worn previously. Muslin gowns were frequently embroidered in white or woven with a gold or silver thread for evening or Court dress. Ribbon trimming was also fashionable. In 1813 Jane Austen

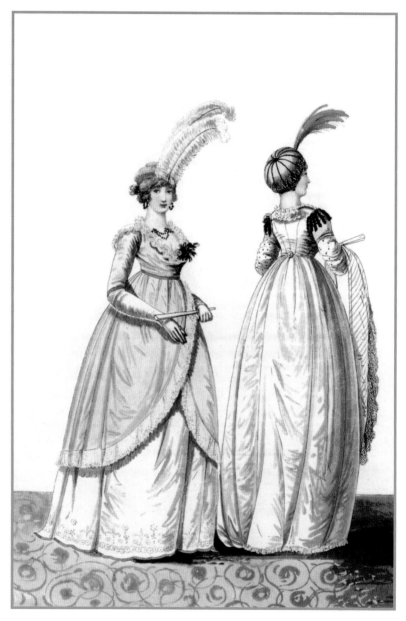

Niklaus von Heideloff, *The Gallery of Fashion*, May 1799

wrote: ' My Gown is to be trimmed everywhere with white ribbon plaited on, somehow or other.'[41] A year later she wrote, 'I have determined to trim my lilac sarsenet with black sattin ribbon ... Ribbon trimmings are all the fashion at Bath ...' Further on in the letter she says: 'I have been ruining myself in black sattin ribbon with a proper perl edge; & now I am trying to draw it up into kind of Roses, instead of putting it in plain double plaits.'[42]

Another popular trimming was bugle beads which were tube-shaped glass beads, usually black. In London in 1811 she mentions buying some bugle trimming at 2/4d[43] and wearing a band of it on her head like the border to her gown.[44] Mrs Elton in *Emma* was very concerned with the decoration of her dress. 'How do you like my gown? How do you like my trimming!' she asked and on another occasion, 'I do not know whether it is not over-trimmed; I have the greatest dislike to the idea of being over-trimmed – quite a horror of finery', but adds a little later, 'I have some notion of putting such a trimming as this to my white and silver poplin.'[45]

Fine white cotton fabrics, especially muslin, were widely worn by the late 1790s but firmer-textured silks, of the type illustrated here, continued in use for gowns and pelisses. Although England had its own silk-weaving industry at Spitalfields in London, many silks were imported from the Continent. There was a ban on French silks during the Napoleonic Wars (not lifted until 1826) but a certain amount of smuggling was carried on.

Shopping

At this period when clothes were made by hand the linen draper, silk mercer and haberdasher where dress fabrics and trimming could be purchased were among the most important shops. Ford's was an imaginary linen draper's where everyone shopped in *Emma* but Jane Austen's letters also give a vivid picture of some of the smart London establishments she visited, such as Grafton House (probably the premises of the drapers Wilding and Kent at the corner of Grafton Street and 164 New Bond Street), Layton and Shear's, mercers of 11 Henrietta Street, Covent Garden and Crook, Son and Besford's a Pall Mall haberdashers and hosiers (which was also patronised by the royal family).[46] In April 1811 she wrote: 'We set off immediately after breakfast & must have reached Grafton House by 1/2 past 11 –, but when we entered the Shop, the whole Counter was thronged, & we waited *full* half an hour before we cd be attended to.'[47]

A typical Bath milliner's shop is illustrated here, selling different fabrics (listed on the drawers at the back). Two ladies examine a length of lace or ribbon. As a fashionable holiday resort, Bath had excellent shops. Many visitors waited until their arrival before buying new clothes for their stay (unlike today when it is usual to stock up before going on holiday). In *Northanger Abbey*, Catherine Morland and Mrs Allen did not go to the Bath Assembly Rooms until they had had an opportunity to find out what was being worn, had made some purchases and Catherine had had her hair 'cut and dressed by the best hand'.

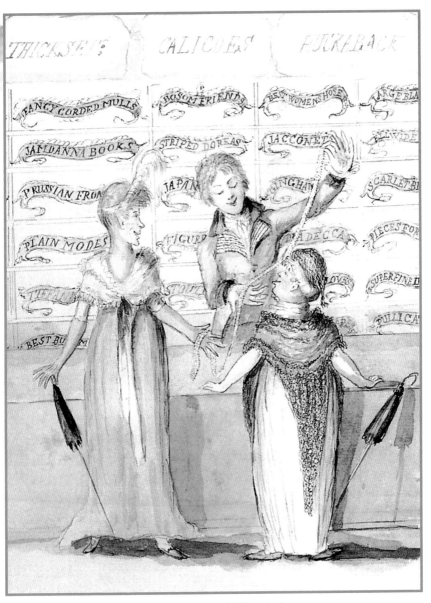

John Sneyd, A Bath Milliner's Shop.
Unpublished illustration to *The New Bath Guide*, c.1810

Two years later she again wrote to Cassandra from London: 'I hope you will receive the Gown tomorrow & may be able with tolerable honesty to say that you like the Colour; – it was bought at Grafton House, where, by going very early, we got immediate attendance, & went on very comfortably. – I only forgot the one particular thing which I had always resolved to buy there – a white silk Handkf – & was therefore obliged to give six shillings for one at Crook & Besford's ... We must have been 3 qrs of an hour at Grafton House, Edward sitting by all the time with wonderful patience. There Fanny bought the Net for Anna's gown, & a beautiful Square veil for herself – The Edging there is very cheap, I was tempted by some, & bought some very nice plaiting Lace at 3-4.'[48] This was a family outing, Edward being her brother, Fanny and Anna, two of her nieces.

Apart from London, Bath was an excellent shopping centre, being a fashionable resort and small enough to walk everywhere with ease. Mrs Allen in *Northanger Abbey* thought Bath a charming place: 'there are so many good shops here. – We are sadly off in the country; not but what we have very good shops in Salisbury, but it is so far to go; – eight miles is a long way ... Now here one can step out of doors and get a thing in five minutes.'[49]

In June 1799 Jane Austen wrote to Cassandra from Bath: 'I saw some Gauzes in a shop in Bath Street yesterday at only 4s a yard, but they were not so good or so pretty as mine.'[50] It is possible that this was the same shop as a haberdasher's called Smith's on the corner of Bath Street where two months later her aunt, the very respectable Mrs Leigh Perrot, was accused of shoplifting. It seems that a piece of white lace was 'accidentally' wrapped in a parcel of purchases she had made with her husband. When the case was eventually brought before the Taunton Assizes the verdict was 'not guilty' and it appears this was a blackmail attempt by the shop. Nevertheless, Mrs Leigh Perrot had been charged with attempted larceny and committed to Ilchester gaol from August 1799 until the trial in March 1800, although she was allowed, with her husband, to live in the jailer's house, rather than the prison. Had she been found guilty the sentence could have been fourteen years transportation or even death.

Dyeing and Cleaning

Women's clothes during this period seem quite frequently to have been dyed either to provide an alternative fashionable colour for a gown or to convert other clothes into mourning. Dyeing was not always successful and in October 1808 Jane asked her sister: 'how is your blue gown? – Mine is all to pieces. – I think there must have been something wrong in the dye, for in places it divided with a Touch. – There was four shillings thrown away; – to be added to my subjects of never failing regret.'[51]

Some dyers also carried out a certain amount of cleaning of clothes. A number of different cleaning agents apart from soap and water were employed, especially for silk and wool fabrics which could not be washed, such as ox-gall, Fullers Earth, French chalk, milk, lemon juice, butter and soda.[52]

The washing of clothes and linen in each household represented a large job which often required extra help from outside. A woman might be employed to come and do the washing or it might be sent out to be done. Commenting on some of the household servants at Steventon in October 1798 Jane Austen remarked: 'Dame Bushell washes for us only one week more, as Sukey has got a place. – John Steevens' wife undertakes our Purification; She does not look as if anything she touched would ever be clean, but who knows?'[53] In *Northanger Abbey*, Catherine Morland, hunting through an old cabinet in the guest bedroom ecstatically discovers what she hopes to be an old and secret manuscript, only to find that: 'an inventory of linen, in coarse and modern characters, seemed all that was before her! If the evidence of sight might be trusted, she held a washing-bill in her hand. She seized another sheet, and saw the same articles with little variation; a third, a fourth, and a fifth, presented nothing new. Shirts, stockings, cravats and waistcoats, faced her in each. Two others, penned by the same hand, marked an expenditure scarcely more interesting, in letters, hair-powder, shoe-string, and breeches-ball [a kind of soap].'[54]

Constant washing of cotton gowns could have poor results and Jane Austen was complaining in September 1796: 'I am sorry to say that my new coloured gown is very much washed out, though I charged everybody to take great care of it.'[55] Catherine Morland is teased by Henry Tilney when he admires her gown but says: 'I do not think it will wash well; I am afraid it will fray.'[56] Muslins were certainly very fragile and liable to tear easily. In *Sense and Sensibility* when Miss Steele meets Elinor Dashwood in Hyde Park she rudely remarks: 'La! if you have not got your spotted muslin on! – I wonder you was not afraid of its being torn!'[57] Miss Steele is felt to be equally ill-bred in her conversation with Marianne Dashwood: 'nothing escaped *her* minute observation and general curiosity; she saw everything, and asked everything; was never easy till she knew the price of every part of Marianne's dress; could have guessed the number of her gowns altogether with better judgement than Marianne herself, and was not without hopes of finding out before they parted, how much her washing cost per week, and how much she had every year to spend upon herself.'[58]

Travelling

When travelling, clothes were normally packed in trunks but in *Northanger Abbey* Catherine Morland also had a few necessary articles packed separately, and on her arrival there she 'was preparing to unpin the linen package, which the chaise-seat had conveyed for her immediate accommodation.'[59] When she was obliged to leave Northanger Abbey at short notice, Eleanor Tilney tried to help with her packing and was 'with more good-will than experience intent upon filling the trunk.'[60] A woman in Eleanor Tilney's social position would have had her packing done by a maid but some ladies took a personal interest in this matter. In *Pride and Prejudice* Lady Catherine de Bourgh, trying to organise Elizabeth Bennet and Maria Lucas, 'inquired minutely into the particulars of their journey, gave them directions as to the best method of packing, and was so urgent on the necessity of placing gowns in the only right way, that Maria thought herself obliged, on her return, to undo all the work of the morning, and pack her trunk afresh.'[61]

Hats and bonnets were carried in a bandbox both when travelling and at home and in *Northanger Abbey* Eleanor Tilney explained the presence of a very heavy old chest in the guest bedroom saying: 'I have not had it moved, because thought it might sometimes be of use in holding hats and bonnets.'[62]

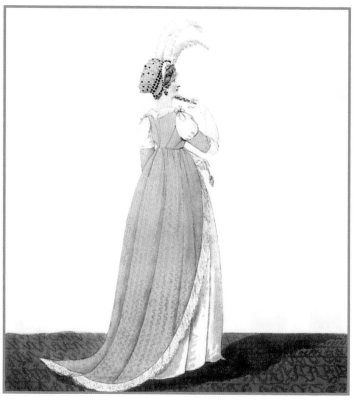

Niklaus von Heideloff, *The Gallery of Fashion*, May 1801

Open-fronted gown of pink fabric edged with lace, worn over a white underskirt or 'petticoat'. Pink and white hat to match, trimmed with black beads and ostrich feathers.

CHAPTER FOUR

Dress for Special Occasions

S OME OF THE special kinds of dress which Jane Austen mentions in both her novels and letters are clothes for mourning or weddings and household liveries.

Mourning

Strict observance of mourning, even for distant relatives, was the rule in the early nineteenth century and the Austens being a large family were often obliged to wear it. A number of references in Jane Austen's letters illustrate the expense involved in reserving special clothes for these occasions, but various expedients such as altering and dyeing other garments were usually found. In October 1808 she wrote to Cassandra from Southampton: 'my mother is preparing mourning for Mrs E. K. [a relative] – she has

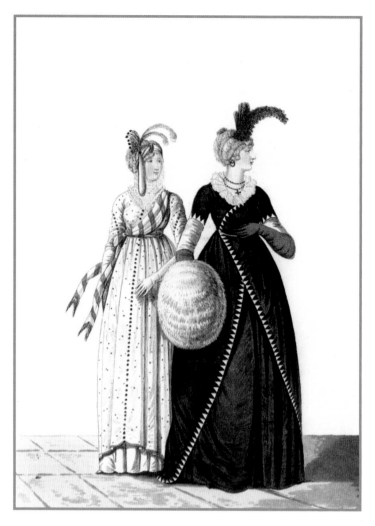

Niklaus von Heideloff, *The Gallery of Fashion*, April 1799

Black clothes were worn for mourning throughout the eighteenth and nineteenth centuries – not only for near and distant relatives but also for members of the royal family. The unrelenting black could be enlivened for evening or formal wear by touches of white, lace, fur, jewellery and feathers.

picked her old silk pelisse to pieces, & means to have it dyed black for a gown – a very interesting scheme.'[1]

A week later, following the sudden and tragic death of their sister-in-law, Elizabeth Austen Knight, she wrote to Cassandra about her own mourning. She was, she said, to be 'in bombazeen and crape, according to what we are told is universal *here*, & which agrees with Martha's previous observation. My mourning, however, will not impoverish me, for by having my velvet Pelisse fresh lined & made up, I am sure I shall have no occasion *this winter* for anything new of that sort. – I take my Cloak for the Lining – & shall send yours on the chance of its doing something of the same for you – tho' I beleive [sic] your Pelisse is in better repair than mine. – *One* Miss Baker makes my gown, & the other my Bonnet, which is to be silk covered with Crape.'[2]

Black bombazine and crape were two materials usually worn for mourning. They were of good quality but their dull finish was considered more suitable than the rich, glossy textures of other silks, satin and velvet. Bombazine was a silk and wool mixture, the wool giving it a matte surface. Black cotton was also worn at times. For example, in January 1801 Jane Austen told her sister: 'You need not endeavour to match my mother's mourning Calico –, she does not mean to make it up any more.'[3]

Crape (as opposed to crepe) was a distinctive mourning fabric much worn throughout the nineteenth century. It was a type of silk gauze with a crimped surface which gave it a dull effect. Crape was used by both men and women as a trimming for outer garments, for hat bands, bonnets, caps and veils.

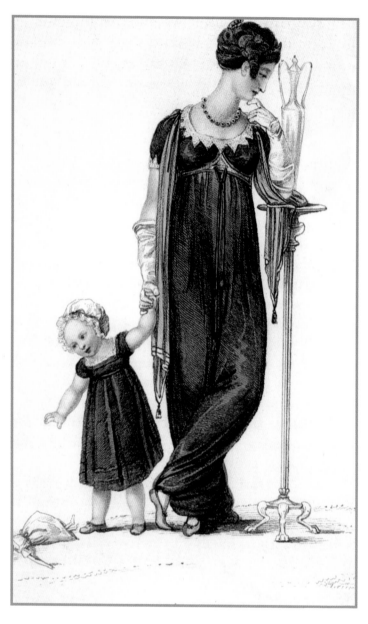

Mourning Dresses, *Ackermann's Repository of Arts*, 1809

It was also usual to observe public mourning for deaths in the royal family and in August 1805 she wrote: 'I suppose everybody will be black for the D. of G. Must we buy lace, or will ribbon do?'⁴ In June 1811 she said she had gone to Alton with her niece Anna and a friend: 'Their business was to provide mourning, against the King's death; & my Mother has had a Bombasin bought for her.'⁵ George III became permanently deranged in this year but did not, in fact, die until 1820. In London in March 1814 she was concerned with the question of whether or not to have a new gown made just at a time when mourning was being observed for the Queen's brother the Duke of MecklenburgStrelitz. 'A grand thought has struck me as to our Gowns. This 6 weeks mourning makes so great a difference that I shall not go to Miss Hare [a milliner in London], till you can come & help chuse yourself; unless you particularly wish the contrary. – It may be hardly worthwhile perhaps to have the Gowns so expensively made up; we may buy a cap or a *veil* instead … Almost everybody was in mourning last night, but my brown gown did very well … I have determined to trim my lilac sarsenet: with black sattin ribbon just as my China crape is, 6d width at bottom, 3d or 4d at top … With this addition

Although the high-waisted muslin dresses of Jane Austen's time are usually illustrated in white or light colours, black dresses for mourning wear also appear in fashion magazines. Mourning did not preclude clothes from being made in the very latest styles or from looking as decorative as possible, once the first phase of deepest mourning had passed. Babies and children were also put into black mourning clothes.

it will be a very successful gown, happy to go anywhere.'[6] Black was, of course, the most usual colour for mourning but as she says, brown on occasion was also acceptable. Second mourning, that is, half mourning worn before the return to normal wear, included lighter colours such as white, grey and lilac trimmed with black.

In *Emma* when Mr Weston's unpleasant sister-in-law dies he resolves 'that his mourning should be as handsome as possible; and his wife sat sighing and moralising over her broad hems, with a commiseration and good sense, true and steady.'[7] Deep hems on linen were another feature of mourning. Men wore crape round their hats as did William Elliot for his first wife who died in 1814; his cousin Elizabeth also wore black ribbons for her.[8]

Weddings

Another occasion for which special clothes were necessary was a wedding, although at this period it was not so much the wedding dress itself as the trousseau which was so important to the bride. The 'wedding

The riding habit was a very practical and versatile garment in the late eighteenth and early nineteenth centuries. Not only was it worn for riding (side saddle) but it was also used for travelling in an open or closed carriage – and for walking. In *Emma*, when Jane Fairfax nearly drowned at Weymouth, Mr Dixon saved her from falling out of the boat by catching hold of her 'habit'. The eighteenth century riding habit was styled in woollen cloth on the lines of the male great coat.

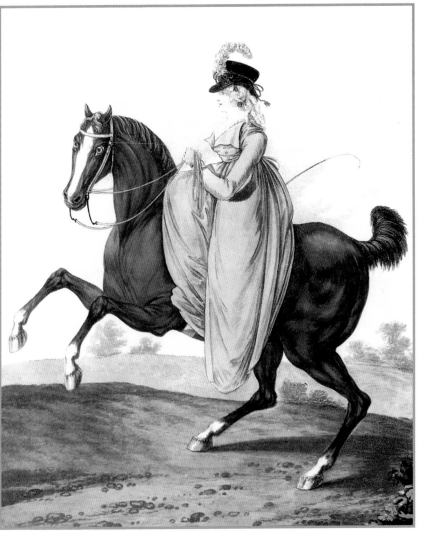

Niklaus von Heideloff, *The Gallery of Fashion*, May 1797

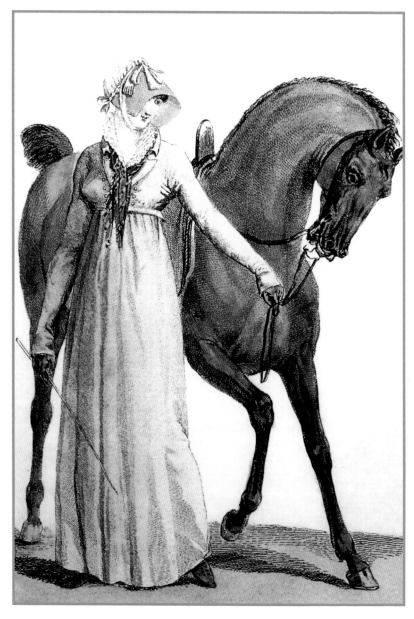

Riding Habit, *Costume Parisien*, 1806

clothes' or trousseau often meant a special visit to London to order and buy from the so-called 'warehouses' (another name for a large shop or emporium) – and large sums of money could be involved. In *Northanger Abbey* Eleanor Tilney's mother had apparently had: 'a very large fortune; and when she married, her father gave her twenty thousand pounds, and five hundred to buy wedding-clothes. Mrs Hughes saw all the clothes after they came from the warehouse.'[9]

In *Pride and Prejudice* when Lydia Bennet eloped and lived with George Wickham for two weeks in London her family were not only shocked by the disgrace of it but were also worried that Wickham might not marry her at all. As far as Lydia's mother was concerned, however, the most important aspect of any marriage were the wedding clothes and so she urged: 'do not let them wait for that, but tell Lydia she shall have as much money as she chooses, to buy them, after they are married'[10]; (but later she goes on to say that Lydia should not 'give any directions about her clothes, till she has seen me, for she does not know which are the best warehouses'[11]. Unfortunately both Lydia and her

Because it was a recognised form of travelling dress, brides often wore riding habits for 'going away' in the early nineteenth century. Lightweight summer versions of the riding habit were made from natural coloured linen or cotton cloth. A short-waisted blouse with a frilled collar (called a 'habit shirt') was worn under the jacket bodice. Very long sleeves, reaching over the knuckles, were a feature of both male and female fashion at this date.

mother were to be disappointed and Mrs Bennet found 'with amazement and horror, that her husband would not advance a guinea to buy clothes for his daughter … She was more alive to the disgrace, which the want of new clothes must reflect on her daughter's nuptials, than to any sense of shame at her eloping and living with Wickham, a fortnight before they took place.'[12]

The propriety of Emma's wedding, on the other hand, could not be questioned, although the author gives us no details: 'the wedding was very much like other weddings, where the parties have no taste for finery or parade.'[13] But Mrs Elton thought it sounded very dull: 'very little white satin, very few lace veils; a most pitiful business.'[14] The lace veils mentioned here in the plural do not refer to the bridal veil but to the fashionable bonnet veils worn by the female guests.

A more detailed description of a wedding – in the Austen family – has been left by Jane Austen's niece Caroline whose half-sister Anna married Benjamin Lefroy on 8 November 1814. 'Weddings', she wrote, 'were then usually very quiet. The old fashion of festivity and publicity had quite gone by, and was universally condemned as showing the bad taste of former generations … I and Anne Lefroy, nine and six years old, wore white frocks and had white ribband on our straw bonnets, which I suppose were new for the occasion.' The dress of the bride was later described by one of her own daughters: it was 'of fine white muslin, and over it a soft silk shawl, white, shot with primrose, with embossed white satin flowers and the delicate yellow tints must have been most becoming to her bright brown hair, hazel eyes, and sunny clear complexion.'[15]

Liveries

A livery was originally a distinctive form of dress worn by the servants of an important person or household so that they might be immediately recognisable in the street. Liveried servants were still employed by many families in Jane Austen's lifetime. A baronet like Sir Walter Elliot in *Persuasion* had his own family livery and we are given some idea of its colour when he surmised that Admiral Croft's weather-beaten face would be 'about as orange as the cuffs and capes of my livery.'[16] Valuing his titled status as he did, Sir Walter Elliot would no doubt have been distressed to hear his cousin and heir presumptive declare that 'if baronetcies were saleable, anybody should have his for fifty pounds, arms and motto, name and livery included.'[17]

A servant's livery would draw attention to his master or household. In *Pride and Prejudice* when Mr Darcy and his sister called to visit Elizabeth Bennet she was warned of their coming by recognising the servant's livery from the window.[18] In *Persuasion* Mary Musgrove failed to notice William Elliot and his servant at Lyme only because they were in mourning. 'I am sure, I should have observed them and the livery too; if the servant had not been in mourning one should have known him by the livery.'[19]

A livery also emphasised the owner's social or financial status. Several other families in Jane Austen's novels have liveried servants. The Tilneys, for example, travelled with 'postilions handsomely liveried'[20] and even the Edwards family in *The Watsons* 'live quite in-style. The door will be opened by a Man in Livery with a powder'd head.'[21]

CHAPTER FIVE

Men's Dress

THE FASHIONS 1775 – 1817

THE MALE SUIT consisted of a coat, waistcoat and knee breeches. The form of these garments remained constant during the eighteenth century but changes were brought about by gradual alterations in cut. There were two main variations of the eighteenth century coat: the more formal version was sloped back at the sides in a curve from the waist; in the 1770s a small standing collar became fashionable. For more informal occasions, for comfort or for sport, the so-called frock coat could be worn (but this style was not the same as the nineteenth century frock coat). The eighteenth century frock coat had an easy cut and fit and also a turned down collar; it was cut away at the sides to form tails which improved the fall of the coat on horseback. In the last decades of the eighteenth century the 'frock' became the more fashionable garment for ordinary wear while the 'coat' was reserved for formal events and then gradually passed out of common use. By the early nineteenth century the style of the frock coat, also known as the riding coat, was varied. Coats could be single or double-breasted, the tails could be cut in horizontally across the waist or gently sloped back at the sides and the lower edge of the tails cut square or rounded.

The waistcoat was cut on similar lines to the coat and was not necessarily sleeveless. At the end of the eighteenth century the shorter, double-breasted waistcoat with a small standing collar became fashionable.

Tight fitting knee breeches were worn during the later eighteenth century but from the 1790s pantaloons were also fashionable. These were a longer, close fitting garment, shaped to the leg and worn with boots. In the early years of the nineteenth century trousers, which were not fitted to the leg, were introduced for informal wear and in time could be worn in the evening as well. Breeches and pantaloons were worn with white or patterned stockings.

The early nineteenth century man's suit could comprise garments of contrasting colours and materials. Fashionable colours for the coat were brown, dark green and dark blue woollen cloth, while breeches and pantaloons tended to be light coloured.

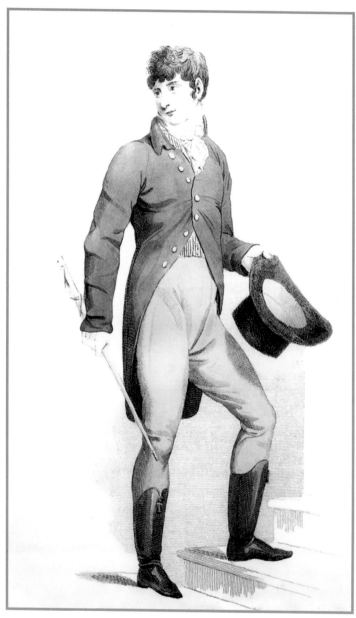

Morning Walking Dress, *Le Beau Monde*, November 1806

Men's Dress in the novels and letters of Jane Austen

There are comparatively few references to male dress in Jane Austen's letters and novels and it is likely that she had only the briefest interest in the subject. Many of her female characters, however, are attracted by men in naval or military uniforms and of course at this period of war, with British victories abroad, the services were both visible and popular. Jane Austen herself had two brothers in the navy.

In *Pride and Prejudice* the younger Misses Bennet were hardly interested in any man who was not in uniform and their mother sympathises with them saying: 'I remember the time when I liked a red coat myself very well ... I thought Colonel Forster looked very becoming the other night at Sir William's in his Regimentals.'[1] In *Mansfield Park* William Price was, 'complete in his Lieutenant's uniform, looking and moving all the taller, firmer, and more graceful for it.'[2]

Early-nineteenth century day wear for men was a smart version of late-eighteenth century riding dress. The morning coat (so-called because a gentleman's normal morning occupation was riding) had the front edges sloped back to form a swallow tail. It was tailored in woollen cloth and was worn with knee breeches or, as here, pantaloons tucked into hussar boots (a fashionable style with curved tops and a tassel at the front). The riding hat with tall, hard crown was now in common use.

Clergymen in the novels did not wear any distinctive form of dress, however. There was nothing in Henry Tilney's attire, for example, to indicate that he was a clergyman when Catherine Morland first met him in *Northanger Abbey*. In *Mansfield Park* Mary Crawford said of Edmund Bertram: 'luckily there is no distinction of dress now-a-days to tell tales'[3] although Edmund himself said that 'a clergyman cannot be high in state or fashion. He must not head mobs, or set the ton in dress.'[4]

One of Jane Austen's rare comments on male dress in her letters concerned a friend, Tom Lefroy, who had 'one fault, which time will, I trust, entirely remove – it is that his morning coat is a great deal too light. He is a very great admirer of Tom Jones, and therefore wears the same coloured clothes, I imagine which *he* did when he was wounded.'[5] Her amusement refers to an incident in Henry Fielding's novel *Tom Jones* (published in 1749): 'as soon as the sergeant was departed, Jones rose from his bed, and dressed himself entirely, putting on even his coat, which, as its colour was white, showed very visibly the streams of blood which flowed down it.'[6] Both Bingley and Wickham, fashionable young men in *Pride and Prejudice*, wore blue coats.[7]

In *Sense and Sensibility* John Willoughby resented the fact that Colonel Brandon 'has more money than he can spend, more time than he knows how to employ, and two new coats every year.'[8] Colonel Brandon was not, at first, much liked by Marianne Dashwood either, as he wore a flannel waistcoat. She imagined him to be very old (although he was only thirty-five) and the flannel waistcoat confirmed her opinion. It was a garment which she 'invariably connected with aches, cramps, rheumatisms, and every species of ailment that can afflict the old and feeble.'[9] Jane Austen herself rather disliked flannel for she wrote in 1798: 'I gave 2s 3d a yard for my flannel, and I fancy it is not very good, but it is so disgraceful and contemptible an article in itself that its being comparatively good or bad is of little importance.'[10]

Marianne's first impressions of John Willoughby, on the other hand, were that: 'his name was good, his residence was their favourite village, and she soon found out that of all manly dresses a shooting jacket was the most becoming.'[11] A shooting-jacket was an informal jacket or coat for sporting wear.

The great coat was a large, loose overcoat reaching to below the knee and having one or more broad falling collars known as capes. Great coats were in common use especially for travelling; they were practical but were also rather cumbersome. In *Northanger Abbey* when it rained one morning in Bath Mrs Allen remarked: 'I hope Mr Allen will put on his great coat when he goes, but I dare say he will not, for he had rather do anything in the world than walk out in a great coat; I wonder he should dislike it, it must be so comfortable.'[12] When travelling with the Tilneys, Catherine thought that the innumerable capes of Henry's great coat 'looked so becomingly important!'[13]

Men's shirts and cravats were usually made by their families at home. Shirts were made of linen, often Irish. In January 1799 Jane Austen told Cassandra: 'when you come home you will have some shirts to make up for Charles [their brother]. Mrs Davies frightened him into buying a piece of Irish [linen] when we were in

Basingstoke.'[14] The following year she wrote: 'I have heard from Charles, & am to send his shirts by half dozens as they are finished; one sett will go next week.'[15] Like Jane Austen, Fanny Price in *Mansfield Park* was kept busy at home making linen for her brother before he went away to sea: 'by working early and late, with perseverance and great dispatch, she did so much that the boy was shipped off at last, with more than half his linen ready.'[16] Catherine Morland on the other hand was not so diligent on her brother's behalf and her mother remarked: 'I do not know when poor Richard's cravats would be done if he had no friend but you.'[17] The cravat was a large triangle or square of muslin, lawn or silk folded crosswise into a band which was then wrapped round the neck with the long ends brought to the front and tied with a knot or bow.

Accessories

Hats: On the head both hats with flat crowns and broad brims and those with moderately tall crowns and medium brims were fashionable at the turn of the century. For the evening, a folding 'opera hat', a bicorne or semicircular-shaped hat could be tucked under the arm when not being worn (and was also known as a *chapeau bras*).

Footwear: Leather jackboots were worn for riding, walking or travelling and reached to just below the knee. Gaiters to cover the leg could also be worn for riding and they were usually made of leather, fastening along the outside of the leg. At one point in *Emma*, Mr Knightley 'was hard at work upon the lower button of his thick leather gaiters'.[18] Indoors, flat leather shoes fastening either with decorative buckles or tie laces were worn.

Gloves: Gloves could be bought at a linendraper's shop like Ford's, the principal shop of the small town in *Emma*. While visiting Highbury, Frank Churchill, in the company of Emma, finds that they are approaching Ford's and he exclaims: 'ha! this must be the very shop that everybody attends every day of their lives, as my father informs me. He comes to Highbury himself, he says, six days out of the seven, and has always business at Ford's. If it be not inconvenient to you, pray let us go in, that I may prove myself to belong to the place, to be a true citizen of Highbury. I must buy something at Ford's ... I dare say they sell gloves.' 'Oh! yes, gloves and everything.' They go inside and soon see 'the sleek, well-tied parcels of "Men's Beavers" and "York Tan"' being brought down and displayed on the counter.[19] These were two kinds of men's gloves worn at the time. 'York Tan' gloves (for both men and women) were a particular type of buff-coloured suede. White gloves for the evening were also worn by men and women. In *The Watsons* the little boy, Charles Blake, dancing at his first ball was provided with his gloves and charged to keep them on.[20]

Jewellery: Additional accessories to men's dress mentioned by Jane Austen include jewellery and ornaments. For example, there was the toothpick-case which the fashionable Robert Ferrars in *Sense and Sensibility* spent so long in choosing at Gray's the jeweller in London. 'He was giving orders for a toothpick-case

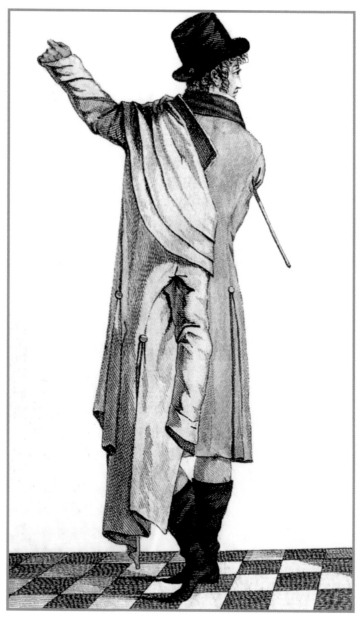

Mise d'un Elégant, *Costume Parisien*, 1779/1800

for himself, and till its size, shape and ornaments were determined, all of which, after examining and debating for a quarter of an hour over every toothpick-case in the shop, were finally arranged by his own inventive fancy ... At last the affair was decided. The ivory, the gold, and the pearls, all received their appointment, and the gentleman having named the last day on which his existence could be continued without the possession of the toothpick-case, drew on his gloves with leisurely care, and ... walked off with an happy air of real conceit and affected indifference.'[21]

It is interesting to see that his serious and much less fashionable brother, Edward, should wear a rather conspicuous piece of jewellery in the form of a ring enclosing a lock of a lady's hair; the ring plays an important part in the plot of *Sense and Sensibility*. During the eighteenth and nineteenth centuries it was popular to wear jewellery made of or containing the hair of a loved friend or relation. The hair was often intricately plaited and set in a brooch, locket or ring, sometimes surrounded by pearls or stones. Miniatures could also be framed at the back with a lock of the sitter's hair. Edward Ferrars' ring was the cause for

The great coat, tailored in heavy, closely-woven woollen cloth (making it both warm and almost impermeable in the days before waterproofing was invented) was essential for coach travel. Multiple shoulder capes gave additional protection in inclement weather. The innumerable capes of Henry Tilney's great coat 'looked so becomingly important', thought Catherine Morland in *Northanger Abbey*.

misunderstanding. Elinor Dashwood, who was in love with Edward, thought the hair it contained was her own and felt confident of his affection because of 'that flattering proof of it which he constantly wore round his finger.'[22] Her rival, Lucy Steele, however, tells her later, 'I gave him a lock of my hair set in a ring … that was some comfort to him, he said, but not equal to a picture.'[23] Two brooches containing the hair of Jane Austen and her father may still be seen in Jane Austen's house at Chawton.

Watches were very fashionable and were carried in the fob pocket of either the breeches or the waistcoat.

Hairdressing: The period of Jane Austen's lifetime saw several changes in the fashion of men's hairdressing. During the last quarter of the eighteenth century men were still wearing wigs or dressing their own hair with powder, but the fashion gradually discontinued and younger men began wearing their own hair cut short. Older and more conservative men still clung to the habit of using powder and there are several references to it in the novels.

In *The Watsons* Mrs Robert Watson scolds her husband for his appearance on the evening of their arrival to stay with their relations: 'you have not put any fresh powder in your hair.' 'No,' he replies, ' – I do not intend it. – I think there is powder enough in my hair for my wife and sisters.' 'Indeed, you ought to make some alteration in your dress before dinner when you are out visiting, though you do not at home.' 'Nonsense' he returns, but a short while later he is overheard telling another guest: 'you cannot be more in deshabille than myself. – We got here so late; that I had not time even to put a little fresh powder in my hair.'[24]

Sir Walter Elliot in *Persuasion* had little respect for Admiral Baldwin's appearance and his head, he said, was only 'nine grey hairs of a side and nothing but a dab of powder at top.'[25] Hair powder (finely ground starch or wheat flour) was usually white but it could be tinted grey, blue or flaxen. It was puffed on with a blower so a powdering jacket or gown, to protect the clothes when the hair was being dressed, could be worn. In *Pride and Prejudice* Mr Bennet threatened to 'sit in my library, in my nightcap and powdering gown, and give as much trouble as I can.'[26] Throughout the eighteenth century the nightcap was worn both in bed and about the house when the wig was removed.

By the beginning of the nineteenth century it was the fashion for men to cut their hair short and it was carefully layered to give a much more natural and informal appearance. The simplicity of the style was nevertheless deceptive; the cut was sophisticated and probably needed frequent attention. Young men like Frank Churchill no doubt took time and trouble over their appearance but 'Emma's very good opinion of Frank Churchill was a little shaken . . . by hearing that he was gone off to London, merely to have his hair cut. A sudden freak seemed to have seized him at breakfast, and he had sent for a chaise and set off, intending to return to dinner, but with no more important view that appeared than having his hair cut. There was certainly no harm in his travelling sixteen miles twice over on such an errand; but there was an air of foppery and nonsense in it which she could not approve ... He came back, had

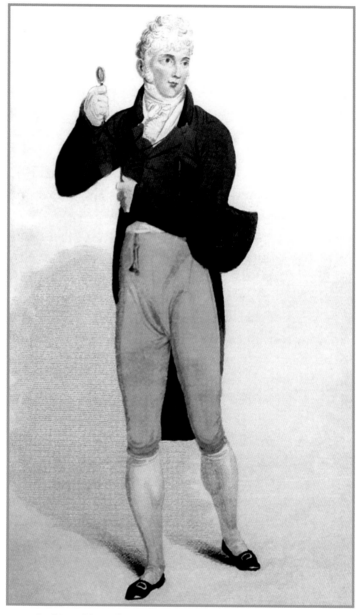

Fashionable Full Dress, *Le Beau Monde*, November 1806

had his hair cut, and laughed at himself with a very good grace, but without seeming really at all ashamed at what he had done. He had no reason to wish his hair longer, to conceal any confusion of face.'[27] Of course, we the readers know that the haircut was merely a pretext and the visit to London was for a secret errand; but it shows that it was thought possible if not very commendable to travel over thirty miles in one day to have a haircut. Well might Frank Churchill have cared about his appearance when some men like Sir Walter Elliot in *Persuasion* were so highly critical. After meeting Admiral Croft Sir Walter felt that 'if his own man might have had the arranging of his hair, he should not be ashamed of being seen with him anywhere.'[28]

As with most new fashions, short unpowdered hair was not welcomed immediately by everyone, and referring to two of her brothers in January 1799 Jane Austen wrote: 'I thought Edward would not approve

For the evening, the more formal 'dress' coat was worn. This coat also had its origins in the eighteenth-century riding coat but the front was cut in straight across the waist and was usually double-breasted. Often made in dark blue cloth with a black velvet collar and gilt buttons, it was worn with a light-coloured waistcoat, breeches, silk stockings and buckled shoes. Although most men no longer wore wigs and had their own hair cut short, powder might still be worn on formal occasions. A semi-circular, folding bicorne hat, white gloves and a monocle were usual accessories to men's evening dress at this date.

of Charles being a crop.'[29] Wigs continued to be worn by some men and in August 1814 she wrote: 'my Brother [James] and Edw'd arrived last night ... Their business is about Teeth & Wigs'.[30] James (born 1765) and Edward (born 1767) were her older brothers and by this date were in their late forties so were perhaps more old-fashioned in their approach to hairdressing.

Extreme personal vanity was the object of Jane Austen's satire with Sir Walter Elliot and, in a middle-aged man, she makes it appear all the more ridiculous. When Admiral Croft rents a house from him he is astounded at Sir Walter's room: 'I should think he must be rather a dressy man for his time of life. – Such a number of looking-glasses! oh, Lord! There was no getting away from oneself. So I got Sophy to lend me a hand, and we soon shifted their quarters; and now I am quite snug, with my little shaving glass in one corner, and another great thing that I never go near.'[31]

CHAPTER SIX

Needlework

A PART FROM THE needlework which most women carried out in the way of making, altering or mending clothes for themselves and for others, there were other forms of handwork which were common or popular pastimes. Needlework usually involved either plain sewing – for example, making or repairing underclothes and household linen – or fine work, in the way of embroidery for decoration and pleasure.

Jane Austen was herself an accomplished needlewoman and her nephew Edward Austen-Leigh was to write in 1870 that 'her needlework both plain and ornamental was excellent, and she might almost have put a sewing machine to shame. She was considered especially great in satin stitch. She spent much time in these occupations, and some of her merriest talk was over clothes which she and her companions were making, sometimes for themselves, and sometimes for the poor.'[1] She herself would not have disclaimed this; in September 1796 she wrote to her sister Cassandra: 'we are very busy making Edward's [their brother] shirts, and I am proud to say that I am the neatest worker of the party.'[2] She was good with her hands in every way and she enjoyed sewing. In December 1808 she told her sister 'I wish I *could* help you in your Needlework, I have two hands & a new Thimble that lead a very easy life.'[3]

Her niece Caroline Austen also remembered that 'she was fond of work and she was a great adept at overcast and satin-stitch – the peculiar delight of that day.'[4] There is a reference to this in one of her letters: her nephew William had worked a footstool for Mrs Austen (his grandmother) but, she says, 'we shall never have the heart to put our feet upon it. – I beleive [sic] I must work a muslin cover in sattin stitch, to keep it from the dirt.'[5] Several pieces of her needlework still survive and may be seen at her house in Chawton; these include a white Indian muslin scarf or shawl embroidered in white cotton in satin stitch. It is made in two pieces joined by a piece of lace insertion at the centre seam. The design consists of small crosses joined by white lines to form an all-over trellis pattern.

Another example of Jane Austen's work is a white lawn pocket handkerchief with a different embroidered motif in each corner, one of which contains the initials *CA.* The handkerchief was made for her sister Cassandra and is a fine example of the delicate white embroidery which was fashionable at the end of the eighteenth and in the early nineteenth centuries.

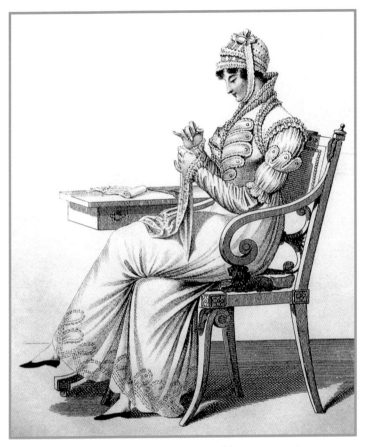

Morning Dress, *La Belle Assemblée*, June 1812

Needlework was the one accomplishment considered necessary for women of every social class to acquire. Sewing skills were learned at an early age and most women were able to mend and alter, if not make, their own clothes. It was also expected of well-to-do ladies to make clothes for the poor. 'I wish *I could* help you in your Needlework,' wrote Jane Austen to her sister Cassandra in 1808. 'I have two hands & a new Thimble that lead a very easy life.'

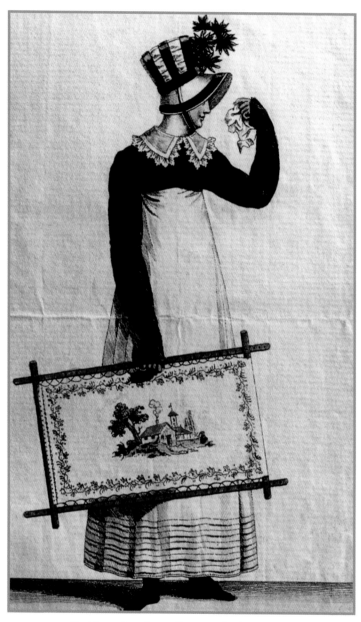

Fashion plate from *Costume Parisien*, 1814

Embroidery

The white muslin dresses which were worn at this period were often decorated with fine white embroidery on the bodice, sleeves, centre panel of the skirt or round the hem. Many of the designs such as the Greek Key pattern were inspired by the neo-classical decoration fashionable in all the arts at this time. Contemporary magazines such as the *Lady's Monthly Museum* published embroidery patterns to be worked on gowns, pelisses or other dress accessories.[6]

Embroidery in coloured silks was also popular especially in the form of needlework pictures. Landscapes, biblical or historical scenes were depicted in silk embroidery on silk or paper and the faces of figures were often drawn and tinted in water-colour. In *Sense and Sensibility,* for example, over the mantelpiece in Charlotte Palmer's bedroom there 'still hung a landscape in coloured silks of her performance, in proof of her having spent seven years at a great school in town to some effect'[7] and Mrs Goddard's neat parlour in *Emma* was 'hung round with fancy-work.'[8]

A fashionable lady, dressed in a satin bonnet and dark blue velvet spencer over a white, flounced gown, carries a piece of embroidery being worked on a frame. In *Sense and Sensibility*, Charlotte Palmer's 'landscape in coloured silks' was probably embroidered in this way.

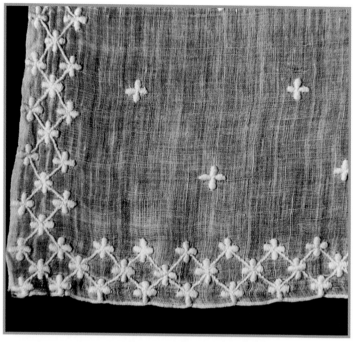

Detail of a white muslin scarf worked in satin stitch by Jane Austen
Jane Austen's House, Chawton

Jane Austen's needlework 'both plain and ornamental was excellent, and she might almost have put a sewing machine to shame' wrote her nephew in 1870. 'She was considered especially great in satin stitch.' Satin stitch is a simple, overcast stitch often used to fill in outlines of motifs such as leaves and petals. The threads, when worked perfectly flat and close together, create a smooth, satin-like effect. This scarf is typical of the light, open-weave muslins fashionable at the turn of the nineteenth century. Fine white embroidery in delicate patterns could add interest and decoration to plain cotton fabrics.

Needlework was, of course, considered to be one of the female accomplishments and most girls began to learn at an early age. Henry Tilney told Catherine Morland in *Northanger Abbey:* 'I had entered on my studies at Oxford, while you were a good little girl working your sampler at home!'[9] (and this would have been when she was about ten years old).

In Jane Austen's novels her characters, both young and old, spend part of each day at their needlework. In *Emma* Jane Fairfax commented to Mrs Bates 'I am sure, grandmama, you must have had very strong eyes to see as you do – and so much fine work as you have done too!'[10] In many cases, to be employed with some kind of work could be both a relief from conversation or provide a topic to discuss. In *Pride and Prejudice* the managing Lady Catherine de Bourgh visiting Charlotte Collins and Elizabeth Bennet 'examined into their employments, looked at their work, and advised them to do it differently.'[11] Later in the novel Elizabeth, confused at receiving a visit from Mr Darcy, 'sat down again to her work, with an eagerness which it did not often command.'[12]

Some of Jane Austen's characters are better at needlework than others. Lady Bertram in *Mansfield Park* was 'a woman who spent her days in sitting nicely dressed on a sofa, doing some long piece of needlework, of little use and no beauty'[13] and, in fact, did not even manage to do it very successfully without constant assistance from her niece Fanny who on several occasions, we read, was 'close beside her arranging her work', 'getting through the few difficulties of her work for her', or 'endeavouring to put her aunt's evening work in such a state as to prevent her being missed.'[14] Julia Bertram doubtless took after her mother because there was relegated to the school-room 'a faded footstool of Julia's work, too ill done for the drawing-room.'[15] As already mentioned, Jane Austen's nephew William had also worked a footstool and this was probably canvas embroidery in tent or cross stitch. 'I long to know what his colours are', she wrote, '– I guess greens and purples.'[16]

Canvas Work

Silk or wool embroidery on a canvas ground had been popular for several centuries for household furnishings such as hangings, coverings, rugs or bed valances and this is probably what is meant by the term 'carpet work' mentioned in several of the novels. It is most unlikely that any of Jane Austen's characters were employing turkeywork techniques and making pile rugs or carpets. It is interesting to note that Mary Delany some fifty years earlier wrote that 'at candlelight cross stitch and reading gather us together. My candlelight work is finishing a carpet in double cross stitch on very coarse canvas to go round my bed.'[17] Lady Bertram had done a great deal of carpet work;[18] and Mrs Jennings was busily employed with it, making a rug (which was probably for the side of her bed although hearth rugs were known by this date);[19] and Emma announced that 'if I give up music, I shall take to carpet-work.'[20]

Tambour Work

Another form of embroidery which reached its height of popularity at the end of the eighteenth century was tambour work. The embroidery was worked on a frame with a fine hook which passed through the fabric and made a series of chain stitches. The work could be done quickly and was effective on lightweight fabrics such as muslin. The frame was circular, mounted on a wooden stand but later a rectangular frame was devised to enable much larger areas to be covered at a time. There is a reference to Mrs Grant's tambour frame in *Mansfield Park*[21] and mention of Catherine Morland's tamboured muslin dress in *Northanger Abbey*.[22]

Patchwork

A further, notable example of Jane Austen's own handwork is the patchwork quilt made by herself, her mother and her sister in the early years of the nineteenth century and which is now on display at her house in Chawton. In May 1811 Jane wrote to Cassandra asking 'have you remembered to collect peices [sic] for the Patchwork? – We are now at a standstill.'[23] The quilt has a deep border of lozenge-shaped, coloured chintz patches and the large, central motif is of floral-patterned chintz surrounded by lozenges outlined in black and white spotted cotton patches.

Apart from embroidery or plain needlework many women also practised the techniques of knotting, netting and knitting to make various accessories for dress or furnishings.

Knotting

Knotting was a popular eighteenth-century craft. Linen, cotton, silk or woollen thread was knotted at regular intervals by means of an oval shuttle (similar to the later tatting shuttle) to form a narrow trimming – the knots resembling a string of small beads. This could be 'laid and couched' (that is placed and sewn onto a piece of fabric) as part of an embroidered decoration or used in short lengths for fringes. One of Jane Austen's nephews, Frank, who was clever with his hands was fond of knotting fringe for curtains when he was a boy and Lady Bertram in *Mansfield Park* apparently made many yards of it.[24] Jane and Cassandra Austen also knotted. In October 1798 Jane wrote from Steventon that at Mrs Ryder's shop there was 'scarcely any netting silk; but Miss Wood, as usual, is going to town very soon, & will lay in a fresh stock.'[25] A few months later in January 1799 she remarked: 'You quite abash me by your progress in notting, for I am still without silk. You must get me some in town or in Canterbury; it should be finer than yours.'[26]

Netting

Netting, also with linen, cotton, silk or wool thread was done with special shuttles (or needles) and gauges to produce a mesh of varying density. It was one of the few drawing-room occupations which were permitted to men and from the evidence of contemporary literature it appears they would often make cherry nets or other nets for use in the garden. Jane Austen's young nephews, at Godmersham Park, she wrote in 1813, 'amuse themselves very comfortably in the Even'g – by netting; they are each about a rabbit net';[27] and Captain Harville in *Persuasion* like many sailors made fishing nets; he also 'fashioned needlework netting-needles and pins with improvements.'[28]

During the last years of the eighteenth century it was the fashion for women to net certain garments – a Miss Debary, Jane Austen wrote in November 1798, 'is netting herself a gown in worsteds'[29] and Isabella Thorpe's friend, Miss Andrews, in *Northanger Abbey* was 'netting herself the sweetest cloak you can conceive.'[30] Catherine Morland also netted and at one point she was 'anxious to be assured of Isabella's having matched some fine netting-cotton' for her[31] but she did not seem to be particularly enthusiastic about any kind of needlework as a little earlier 'the nettingbox, just leisurely drawn forth, was closed with joyful haste.'[32] Netting tools and the work in hand were kept in a special box or case. Most women at this time would have had a netting-box as well as a work-basket for their sewing and, in *Mansfield Park*, in Fanny's room 'the table between the windows was covered with work-boxes and nettingboxes, which had been given her at different times, principally by Tom' (her cousin).[33]

Making purses, in the eighteenth and nineteenth centuries was an important branch of domestic needlework and most of the eighteenth century purses were netted in silk. Later, many were knitted, often with beads or crocheted (crochet being introduced during the first quarter of the nineteenth century). In *Pride and Prejudice* Mr Bingley was impressed that all young ladies were able to 'paint tables, cover skreens

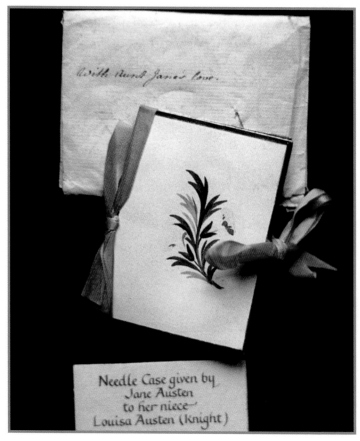

Needle case given to Jane Austen's niece
Jane Austen's House, Chawton

This delicately made and painted needle case is accompanied by a note in Jane Austen's handwriting: 'With Aunt Jane's love'. As well as sewing, ladies often made needlework tools of this kind – usually as gifts, but sometimes to earn a little money. Anne Elliot's friend, Mrs Smith, in *Persuasion* sold 'these little thread-cases, pin-cushions and card-races, which you always find me so busy about' to eke out a living.

and net purses', but Mr Darcy thought it ridiculous that a woman should be considered 'accomplished' simply because she could do these things. 'The word', he said 'is applied to many a woman who deserves it no otherwise than by netting a purse, or covering a skreen.'[34]

Knitting

A certain amount of knitting was also done. Jane Fairfax, in *Emma*, knitted garters for her grandmother[35] and Mrs Smith in *Persuasion* had been taught to knit when she was recovering from a serious illness;[36] but on the whole, knitting at this time appears to be a handcraft associated with the elderly. Jane Fairfax's grandmother, Mrs Bates, for example, was a 'quiet and neat old lady', who with her knitting was seated in the warmest corner',[37] and Jane Austen's mother, she wrote in 1813, 'finds great amusement in the glove-knitting; when this pair is finished, she means to knit another, & at present wants no other work.'[38] Mrs Austen also seems to have knitted rugs and Jane wrote to her sister in 1807: 'Martha's rug is just finished, & looks well, tho' not quite so well as I had hoped. I see no fault in the Border, but the Middle is dingy. – My Mother desires me to say that she will knit one for you, as soon as you return to chuse the colours & pattern.'[39]

Lace

Although few ladies appear to have made lace at home at this time it was fashionable as a dress material or trimming and very highly valued. Machine-made lace began to be produced during the last decades of the eighteenth century. In 1799 Jane Austen bought a cloak in Bath which cost her two pounds. She wrote to Cassandra: 'My Cloak is come home, and here follows the pattern of its lace. – If you do not think it wide enough, I can give 3d a yard more for yours, & not go beyond the two Guineas, for my Cloak altogether does not cost quite two pounds. – I like it very much …'[40]

Lace designs altered with the fashions in dress and by the end of the eighteenth century the patterns showed a popularity for smaller sprigs of flowers scattered over the fine net background. These more delicate designs suited the lighter muslin gowns which were being worn.

Jane also purchased a veil for their sister-in-law, Mary, 'a black Lace one for 16 shillings.'[41] In 1800 Cassandra bought a cloak for Jane in London and Jane wrote to her: 'My Cloak came on tuesday, & tho' I expected a good deal, the beauty of the lace astonished me. – It is too handsome to be worn, almost too handsome to be looked at.'[42] Mrs Allen in *Northanger Abbey* valued her own lace and was glad to see that 'the lace on Mrs Thorpe's pelisse was not half so handsome as that on her own'[43] and when she returned home to Fullerton she told Catherine: 'only think, my dear, of my having got that frightful rent in my best Mechlin so charmingly mended, before I left Bath, that one can hardly see where it was.'[44] Mrs Elton in *Emma* also had a high regard for lace and she herself was as elegant as lace and pearls could make her'.[45] She considered Emma's wedding to be a very poor affair with 'very little white satin, very few lace veils.'[46]

Needlework Tools

Few of Jane Austen's own needlework tools survive but there are in existence some which she made for other people. One is a small needle-book on display in her house at Chawton, delicately made and painted for her niece Louisa and accompanied by a note in her own handwriting 'with Aunt Jane's love'. Her nephew Edward Austen-Leigh also recalled in 1870 that 'there still remains a curious specimen of her needlework made for a sister-in-law, my mother. In a very small bag is deposited a little rolled up housewife [needlework case], furnished with minikin needles and fine thread. In the housewife is a tiny pocket, and in the pocket is enclosed a slip of paper, on which, written as with a crow quill, are these lines:

> This little bag, I hope will prove
> To be not vainly made;
> For should you thread and needles want,
> It will afford you aid.
>
> And as we are about to part,
> 'T will serve another end:
> For when you look upon this bag,
> You'll recollect your friend.

'It is the kind of article that some benevolent fairy might be supposed to give as a reward to a diligent little girl. The whole is of flowered silk, and having been never used and carefully preserved it is as fresh and bright as when it was first made seventy years ago; and shows that the same hand which painted so exquisitely with the pen could work as delicately with the needle.'[47]

References to needlework tools in her novels were no doubt based on familiar objects to Jane Austen. Mrs Smith in *Persuasion* earned a little money by making 'these little thread-cases, pin-cushions and card-racks, which you always find me so busy about.'[48] In *Sense and Sensibility* Lady Dashwood gave each of the Misses Steele 'a needle book, made by some emigrant' [from the Napoleonic Wars].[49] Later, when they are sent away in disgrace, the elder Miss Steele told Elinor Dashwood, 'I was all in a fright for fear your sister should ask us for the housewifes she gave us a day or two before.'[50]

The characters in *Pride and Prejudice* might have had difficulty in defining the truly 'accomplished' woman, but if Caroline Bingley's opinion can be accepted, that 'no one can be really esteemed accomplished, who does not greatly surpass what is usually met with'[51], then without doubt Jane Austen herself was a perfect example. The reminiscences of her relatives, the letters she wrote and her handwork which survives all point to a woman equally well gifted in what were considered the female arts of her time as in the literary world; who took pleasure in her domestic occupations and applied the same standard of perfection to her work of every kind.

Brief Guide to the Textile Terms Used in the Works of Jane Austen

BAIZE: Coarse woollen fabric used for linings, coverings or curtains.

BEAVER: The term covers not only the fabric made of felted wool and fur especially used in the making of hats, but also a thick woollen cloth with a nap-raised finish somewhat resembling plush, used for overcoating.

BOMBAZINE: Bombasin, Bombazin, Bombazeen. Dress material usually made with a silk warp and wool worsted weft in a twill weave; sometimes of cotton and wool worsted or worsted alone. Dyed black, it was frequently worn for mourning because of its dull texture.

CALICO: General name for plain cottons which were heavier than muslin. It was originally imported from India.

CAMBRIC: Very fine white linen, originally made at Cambray in Flanders.

CAMBRIC MUSLIN: This was probably a muslin which resembled cambric, or a fine linen fabric, through the appearance of its yarn and weave.

CHINA CRAPE: A heavier weight than ordinary crape but with the characteristic crinkled surface.

CHINTZ: Cotton cloth printed in various colours and with a glazed surface. It was originally imported from India but by the late eighteenth century was also being produced in large quantities in Europe (Britain included).

CLOTH: Although the term is used for any woven fabric it generally refers to a closely-woven material of fine quality wool.

CRAPE: As a general term this refers to the thin, almost transparent silk gauze fabric with a crimped surface (achieved by the use of a high twist yarn) much used for mourning. A special variant of black crape for mourning was prepared from gummed yarn and had an embossed 'figure' or pattern, which produced a duller, denser texture. (See: D. C. Coleman, *Courtaulds*, Oxford University Press, 1969). Crape spelt with an 'a' usually refers to the black mourning fabric. Crepe with an 'e' is a later spelling denoting a similar fabric with a crinkled surface but made in a variety of colours for general use.

DIMITY: A firm cotton fabric woven with a small raised pattern or stripe. It was usually undyed.

FLANNEL: Plain woollen fabric with a loose weave.

GAUZE: A very thin, almost transparent fabric of silk, cotton or linen distinguished by the twisted thread of its weave.

IRISH: A type of linen, originating from its place of manufacture, Ireland.

JACONET: Jackonet. A thin, soft variety of muslin.

KERSEYMERE: Fine woollen cloth, closely woven, with a twill weave.

LINON: Murray's *New English Dictionary* (1908) defines this as a trade-name for lawn (a kind of fine white linen similar to cambric) and it may possibly have had the same meaning in Jane Austen's period.

MUSLIN: A general term for soft, thin, loosely woven cotton fabrics. The finest muslins traditionally came from India.

NANKIN: Nankeen. A twilled cotton cloth with a natural yellowish brown tint, originally produced in Nanking, China.

NET: A meshed fabric of which the threads may be twisted, plaited, looped or knotted.

PERSIAN: A thin, soft, plain silk often used for linings.

POPLIN: Fabric of silk and wool worsted (or can be made of cotton) with a corded surface.

SARSENET: Sarcenet. A fine, soft silk, usually with a twill weave.

SATIN: Silk fabric with a glossy surface.

STUFF: Plain or twilled woollen fabric woven with long staple fibres.

VELVET: Fabric with a short, dense and smooth piled surface, usually silk (but sometimes of cotton).

WORSTED: A woollen fabric which, in common with stuff, used long staple fibres.

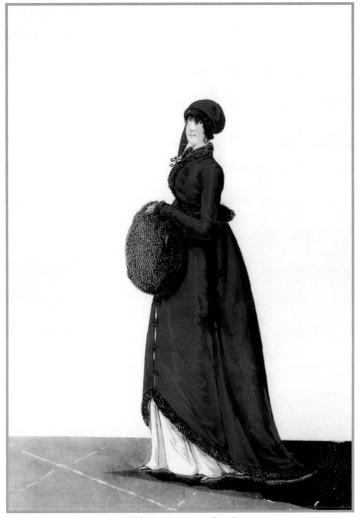

Niklaus von Heideloff, *The Gallery of Fashion*, January 1803

Pelisse (worn over a white gown) and matching cap of crimson silk trimmed with brown fur and cord frogging in the 'hussar' style. Large fur muff to match.

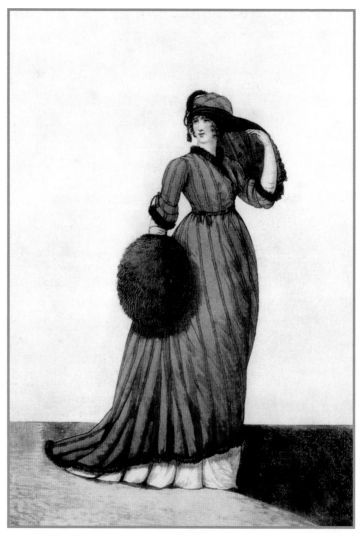

Niklaus von Heideloff, *The Gallery of Fashion*, January 1800

Pelisse of striped pink fabric, trimmed (or possibly lined throughout) with brown fur, with tasselled cap to match. Worn with a black lace veil, cream leather gloves and large brown fur muff.

122

References

The following references to the novels and letters are taken from the Oxford University Press editions listed in the Short Bibliography.

CHAPTER ONE: Jane Austen

1 *Mansfield Park*, p. 254
2 *Northanger Abbey*, pp. 73–4

CHAPTER TWO: Women's Dress

1 *Pride and Prejudice*, p. 139
2 *Pride and Prejudice*, p. 222
3 *Letters*, Friday 2 September 1814
4 *Letters*, Thursday 30 June 1808
5 *Persuasion*, p. 65
6 *Mansfield Park*, p. 395
7 *Pride and Prejudice*, p. 36
8 *Letters*, Monday 24 December 1798
9 *Letters*, Wednesday 9 March 1814
10 *Letters*, Friday 2 September 1814
11 *Pride and Prejudice*, p. 140
12 *Letters*, Tuesday 18 December 1798 and Tuesday 5 May 1801
13 *Minor Works*, 'The Watsons', p. 327
14 *Northanger Abbey*, p. 37
15 *Letters*, Wednesday 15 September 1813
16 *Letters*, Thursday 21 October 1813
17 *Letters*, Sunday 25 November 1798
18 *Letters*, Saturday 25 – Monday 27 October 1800
19 *Letters*, Thursday 18 April 1811
20 *Letters*, Thursday 16 September 1813
21 *Emma*, p. 86
22 *Mansfield Park*, p. 305
23 *Letters*, Sunday 21 April 1805
24 *Northanger Abbey*, p. 28–9
25 *Letters*, Tuesday 18 December 1798. A cawl or caul was the foundation or crown of a bonnet or cap.
26 *Letters*, Tuesday 5 – Wednesday 6 May 1801
27 *Pride and Prejudice*, pp. 219 and 221
28 *Letters*, Sunday 2 June 1799. Note: Jane Austen's parents were married in Walcot Church, Bath in 1764. Her father was buried there in 1805.
29 *Letters*, Tuesday 11 June 1799
30 *Northanger Abbey*, p. 39
31 *Letters*, Tuesday 18 – Wednesday 19 December 1798
32 *Letters*, Tuesday 8 January 1799
33 *Fashions of London and Paris*, February 1804. See also: Anne

Buck, 'The Costume of Jane Austen and her Characters', in *The So-Called Age of Elegance*, Proceedings of the Fourth Annual Conference of the Costume Society, Spring 1970, pp. 36–45

34 *Letters*, Wednesday 15 September and Thursday 16 September 1813

35 *Minor Works*, 'Sanditon', p. 383

36 *Letters*, Friday 9 September 1814

37 *Letters*, Sunday 2 June 1799

38 *Minor Works*, 'The Watsons', p. 347

39 *Mansfield Park*, pp. 360–1

40 *Emma*, p. 127

41 *Emma*, p. 89

42 *Minor Works*, 'The W atsons', p. 345

43 *Persuasion*, p. 135

44 James-Edward Austen-Leigh, *Memoir of Jane Austen*, p. 40

45 *Northanger Abbey*, p. 184

46 *Letters*, Thursday 21 May 1801

47 *Minor Works*, 'Sanditon', p. 381

48 *Persuasion*, p. 177

49 *Letters*, Sunday 24 January 1813

50 *Letters*, Saturday 27 October 1798

51 *Letters*, Thursday 20 May 1813

52 *Letters*, Tuesday 8 – Wednesday 9 January 1799

53 *Mansfield Park*, p. 279

54 *Northanger Abbey*, p. 77

55 *Emma*, p. 453

56 *Pride and Prejudice*, p. 39

57 *Emma*, p. 479

58 *Northanger Abbey*, p. 56

59 *Mansfield Park*, p. 254

60 *Mansfield Park*, p. 258

61 *Mansfield Park*, p. 262

62 *Letters*, Tuesday 26 – Wednesday 27 May 1801

63 *Sense and Sensibility*, p. 220

64 *Sense and Sensibility*, p. 226

65 *Emma*, p. 324

66 *Northanger Abbey*, pp. 68–9

67 *Minor Works*, 'Sanditon', pp. 374 and 390

68 *Pride and Prejudice*, p. 238

69 Caroline Austen, *My Aunt Jane Austen*, p. 5

70 *Letters*, Saturday 1 – Sunday 2 December 1798

71 *Letters*, Saturday 24 August 1805

72 *Letters*, Wednesday 15 – Thursday 16 September 1813

73 *Persuasion*, p. 215

74 *Persuasion*, p. 35

75 *The Bath Chronicle*, 6 January 1814. See also Buck, op. cit.

76 *Persuasion*, pp. 145–6

77 *Northanger Abbey*, p. 223

78 *Letters*, Wednesday 14 – Friday 15 January 1801

79 *Emma*, p. 167

80 *Emma*, p. 270

81 *Northanger Abbey*, pp. 55–6

82 *Emma*, p. 484

83 *Mansfield Park*, p. 272

84 *Northanger Abbey*, p. 74

85 Caroline Austen, *My Aunt Jane Austen*, p. 5

86 *Letters*, Saturday 1 – Sunday 2 December 1798

87 *Pride and Prejudice*, p. 36

CHAPTER THREE: The Making and Care of Clothes

1 *Letters*, Sunday 29 November 1812

2 James-Edward Austen-Leigh, *Memoir of Jane Austen*, p. 178

3 *Letters*, Thursday 18 – Saturday 20 April 1811

4 *Northanger Abbey*, p. 70

5 *Letters*, Monday 24 – Wednesday 26 December 1798

6 *Letters*, Monday 24 – Wednesday 26 December 1798

7 *Mansfield Park*, p. 254

8 *Emma*, p. 9

9 James-Edward Austen-Leigh, *Memoir of Jane Austen*, p. 98

10 *Letters*, Wednesday 9 March 1814

11 *Letters*, Tuesday 26 – Wednesday 27 May 1801

12 For example, *Letters*, Tuesday 5 – Wednesday 6 May 1801

13 *Letters*, Tuesday 17 – Wednesday 18 January 1809

14 *Letters*, Thursday 14 – Friday 15 October 1813

15 *Mansfield Park*, p. 71

16 *Mansfield Park*, p. 166

17 *Northanger Abbey*, pp. 28–9

18 *Letters*, Sunday 25 January 1801

19 *Letters*, Thursday 18 – Saturday 20 April 1811

20 *Letters*, Wednesday 21 – Thursday 22 January 1801

21 *Emma*, p. 235

22 *Sense and Sensibility*, p. 120

23 *Letters*, Wednesday 7 – Thursday 8 January 1807

24 *Letters*, Thursday 23 – Friday 24 September 1813

25 *Letters*, Sunday 2 June 1799

26 James-Edward Austen-Leigh, *Memoir of Jane Austen*, p. 40

27 *Northanger Abbey*, p. 74

28 *Northanger Abbey*, p. 28

29 *Letters*, Tuesday 11 June 1799

30 *Northanger Abbey*, p. 91

31 *Mansfield Park*, p. 222

32 *Letters*, Tuesday 12 – Wednesday 13 May 1801

33 *Northanger Abbey*, p. 104

34 *Letters*, Thursday 21 – Friday 22 May 1801

35 *Mansfield Park*, p. 105–6

36 *Letters*, Sunday 25 January 1801

37 *Northanger Abbey*, p. 218

38 *Letters*, Thursday 15 – Friday 16 September 1796

39 *Northanger Abbey*, p. 28

40 *Letters*, Saturday 1 December 1798 and Thursday 4 February 1813

41 *Letters*, Wednesday 15 and Thursday 16 September 1812

42 *Letters*, Saturday 5 – Tuesday 8 March 1814

43 *Letters*, Thursday 18 – Saturday 20 April 1811

44 *Letters*, Tuesday 30 April 1811

45 *Emma*, p. 302

46 See: Deirdre Le Faye (ed.), *Jane Austen's Letters*, 1995, pp. 514, 544, 608 and Kay Staniland, *In Royal Fashion. The Clothes of Princess Charlotte of Wales and Queen Victoria 1796–1901*, Museum of London, 1997, p. 85

47 *Letters*, Thursday 18 – Saturday 20 April 1811

48 *Letters*, Thursday 16 September 1813

49 Northanger Abbey, p. 29

50 *Letters*, Sunday 2 June 1799

51 *Letters*, Friday 7 – Sunday 9 October 1808

52 See: Alan Mansfield, 'Dyeing and Cleaning Clothes in the late eighteenth and early nineteenth centuries', in *Costume*, 1967–68, pp. 38–43

53 *Letters*, Saturday 27 – Sunday 28 October 1798

54 *Northanger Abbey*, p. 172

55 *Letters*, Thursday 1 September 1796

56 *Northanger Abbey*, p. 28

57 *Sense and Sensibility*, p. 276

58 *Sense and Sensibility*, p. 249

59 *Northanger Abbey*, p. 163

60 *Northanger Abbey*, p. 227

61 *Pride and Prejudice*, pp. 213–14

62 *Northanger Abbey*, p. 165

CHAPTER FOUR:
Dress for Special Occasions

1 *Letters*, Friday 7 – Sunday 9 October 1808

2 *Letters*, Saturday 15 – Sunday 16 October 1808

3 *Letters*, Wednesday 21 – Thursday 22 January 1801

4 *Letters*, Friday 30 August 1805

5 *Letters*, Thursday 6 June 1811

6 *Letters*, Saturday 5 – Tuesday 8 March 1814. For Miss Hare see Deirdre Le Faye (ed.), *Jane Austen's Letters*, p. 532

7 *Emma*, p. 388

8 *Persuasion*, p. 8

9 *Northanger Abbey*, p. 68

10 *Pride and Prejudice*, p. 288

11 *Pride and Prejudice*, p. 288

12 *Pride and Prejudice*, pp. 310–11

13 *Emma*, p. 484

14 *Emma*, p. 484

15 Mary Augusta Austen-Leigh, *Personal Aspects of Jane Austen*, pp. 135–8

16 *Persuasion*, p. 22

17 *Persuasion*, p. 202

18 *Pride and Prejudice*, p. 260

19 *Persuasion*, p. 106

20 *Northanger Abbey*, p. 156

21 *Minor Works*, 'The Watsons', p. 322

CHAPTER FIVE: Men's Dress

1 *Pride and Prejudice*, p. 29

2 *Mansfield Park*, p. 384

3 *Mansfield Park*, p. 416

4 *Mansfield Park*, p. 92

5 *Letters*, Saturday 9 January 1796

6 Henry Fielding, *Tom Jones*, Book 7, ch. 14

7 *Pride and Prejudice*, pp. 9 and 319

8 *Sense and Sensibility*, p. 51

9 *Sense and Sensibility*, p. 38

10 *Letters*, Saturday 27 October 1798

11 *Sense and Sensibility*, p. 43

12 *Northanger Abbey*, p. 83

13 *Northanger Abbey*, p. 157

14 *Letters*, Monday 21 – Wednesday 23 January 1799

15 *Letters*, Saturday 1 November 1800

16 *Mansfield Park*, p. 390

17 *Northanger Abbey*, p. 240

18 *Emma*, p. 287

19 *Emma*, pp. 199–200

20 *Minor Works*, 'The Watsons', p. 331

21 *Sense and Sensibility*, pp. 220–1

22 *Sense and Sensibility*, p. 102

23 *Sense and Sensibility*, p. 135

24 *Minor Works*, 'The Watsons', p. 353 and p. 357

25 *Persuasion*, p. 20

26 *Pride and Prejudice*, p. 300

27 *Emma*, p. 205 and p. 212

28 *Persuasion*, p. 32

29 *Letters*, Monday 21 January 1799

30 *Letters*, Tuesday 23 – Wednesday 24 August 1814

31 *Persuasion*, p. 128

CHAPTER SIX: Needlework

1 James-Edward Austen-Leigh, *Memoir of Jane Austen*, p. 98

2 *Letters*, Thursday 1 September 1796

3 *Letters*, Tuesday 27 – Wednesday 28 December 1808

4 Caroline Austen, *My Aunt Jane Austen*, p. 7

5 *Letters*, Tuesday 17 – Wednesday 18 January 1809

6 *The Lady's Monthly Museum, or Polite Repository of Amusement and Instruction*. By a Society of Ladies, London, 1808

7 *Sense and Sensibility*, p. 160

8 *Emma*, p. 22

9 *Northanger Abbey*, p. 107

10 *Emma*, p. 158

11 *Pride and Prejudice*, p. 169

12 *Pride and Prejudice*, p. 335

13 *Mansfield Park*, p. 19

14 *Mansfield Park*, p. 125, p. 126 and p. 220

15 *Mansfield Park*, p. 152

16 *Letters*, Tuesday 17 – Wednesday 18 January 1809

17 *The Autobiography and Correspondence of Mary Granville, Mrs Delany*, edited by Lady Llanover, 6 vols., 1861–2. Letter to Mrs Dewes, 1757

18 *Mansfield Park*, p. 179

19 *Sense and Sensibility*, p. 181

20 *Emma*, p. 85

21 *Mansfield Park*, p. 65

22 *Northanger Abbey*, p. 73

23 *Letters*, Friday 31 May, 1811

24 *Mansfield Park*, p. 179

25 *Letters*, Saturday 27 October 1798

26 *Letters*, Monday 21 – Wednesday 23

January 1799

27 *Letters*, Monday 11 – Tuesday
   October 1813
28 *Persuasion*, p. 99
29 *Letters*, Sunday 25 November 1798
30 *Northanger Abbey*, p. 40
31 *Northanger Abbey*, p. 201
32 *Northanger Abbey*, p. 176
33 *Mansfield Park*, p. 153
34 *Pride and Prejudice*, p. 39
35 *Emma*, p. 86
36 *Persuasion*, p. 155
37 *Emma*, p. 156
38 *Letters*, Sunday 24 January 1813
39 *Letters*, Sunday 8 – Monday 9

February 1807

40 *Letters*, Sunday 2 June 1799
41 *Letters*, Tuesday 11 June 1799
42 *Letters*, Saturday 1 November 1800
43 *Northanger Abbey*, p. 32
44 *Northanger Abbey*, p. 238
45 *Emma*, p. 292
46 *Emma*, p. 484
47 James-Edward Austen-Leigh,
   Memoir of Jane Austen, p. 98
48 *Persuasion*, p. 155
49 *Sense and Sensibility*, p. 254
50 *Sense and Sensibility*, p. 275
51 *Pride and Prejudice*, p. 39

Short Bibliography

The novels of Jane Austen edited by R. W. Chapman and first published by Oxford University Press 1923:

Sense and Sensibility (1811)

Pride and Prejudice (1813)

Mansfield Park (1814)

Emma (1816)

Northanger Abbey and *Persuasion* (1818)

Volume VI *Minor Works* (first edition, 1954)

Chapman, R. E. (ed.). *Jane Austen's Letters to her Sister Cassandra and Others.* Oxford University Press, 1932; 2nd edn., 1952.

Le Faye, Deidre (ed.). *Jane Austen's Letters.* Oxford University Press, 1995. New edition.

Austen, Caroline. *My Aunt Jane Austen* (1867). Printed for the Jane Austen Society, 1952.

Austen-Leigh, James-Edward. *A Memoir of Jane Austen* (1870). Oxford University Press, 1926.

Austen-Leigh, Mary Augusta. *Personal Aspects of Jane Austen.* London, 1920.